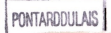
All Creatures

All Creatures

Heartwarming Tales from a Yorkshire Vet

Julian Norton

CORONET

First published in Great Britain in 2021 by Coronet
An Imprint of Hodder & Stoughton
An Hachette UK company

Paperback ISBN 9781529378429
eBook ISBN 9781529378382

Typeset in Electra LH by Palimpsest Book Production Ltd, Falkirk, Stirlingshire

Printed and bound in Great Britain by Clays Ltd, Elcograf S.p.A.

Hodder & Stoughton policy is to use papers that are natural, renewable
and recyclable products and made from wood grown in sustainable forests.
The logging and manufacturing processes are expected to conform
to the environmental regulations of the country of origin.

Hodder & Stoughton Ltd
Carmelite House
50 Victoria Embankment
London EC4Y 0DZ

www.hodder.co.uk
www.hodder.co.uk

To all the creatures I've treated.

In Spite of their diversities
And perversities
Both zoological
And ideological,
They all gathered together
One day, when the weather
Was especially frightful, and decided
It wasn't safe to stay divided
Any longer, and that they should,
For their common good,
(Rather than risk another calamity)
Try Amity.
And that's the day there began to dawn a
Plan they christened UNITED FAUNA

Melville Cane

Contents

Introduction   1

Part 1

Cows   3
Slow Fever and a Journey in the Fog   7
Cast Your Bread   16
Maurice and the Milk Fever   22
Death at Embleton's   30
Extirpating Bertha   36

Part 2

Dogs   49
The Hound of Gormire   52
This Week I have been Mostly
    Sticking my Finger up Dogs' Bottoms   60
Nelly with the Elephant Legs   67
Reel Around the Fountain   73
I Think it's a Bloody Version of . . .   78

Part 3

Pigs   87
All Sorts of Farmers   91
Beetroot Sandwiches   103
Has Anyone Seen our Sow?   112
Certainly not Boaring   119

Part 4

Horses and Donkeys   129
Blossom the Shire Horse
    and Basil the Donkey   132
Cheltenham and York   138
Donkey Sagas   149
Foalings   158

Part 5

Cats   171
Bouncing Cats   174
Sandbeck's First Patient   179
Smokey and the Grass Cuttings   188
The Cat's Bottom   197

Part 6

Sheep and Goats   203
Prolapse!   207
Dilating in the Moonlight   215
Activated Goat   223
Grumpy Farmer?   231

Part 7

Llamas and Alpacas   243
Intensive Cria Unit   246
Alpacas in the Practice   255
Alpacas on the Telly   264
Camelid Calamities   268

Part 8

All Creatures   277
Boris. Luna, Babs and Betty   279
Ferrets   288
The Birds   295
We're All Going to the Zoo Tomorrow   303
The Last Calving?   313

Introduction

Happy animals are all alike, although each type in its own way. A Cocker Spaniel will constantly wag his tail as he dashes about on his morning walk, sniffing and investigating. He's permanently happy, like a child who never stops smiling. The cows in the field next to the spaniel's walk are ruminating placidly, as they digest the last remnants of goodness from the autumn grass. They are not so animated, but are quietly content in their own way. One might make a mooing noise, seeking reassurance from her herd-mates that everything is okay and that is about as excited as a grazing bovine gets, but contentment is the key.

Of course, we don't know what is going on in their heads, because these creatures cannot talk, but maybe they don't need to. Watching a gang of two-week-old piglets play hide-and-seek around the sow as she languishes in the straw, it is impossible not to believe that they are having a lot of fun. Lambs will skip and gambol, with all the energy of youth, in the warmth of late-spring sunshine. It is safe to assume they are happy creatures. A fuzzy kitten, with a stumpy tail pointing skywards, cautiously explores her new surroundings with trepidation but surely also a smile inside. You can almost hear her thoughts: 'Hmm, what's going on over here?'

And a dog, grateful for his veterinary care, lifts his front leg for yet another blood sample. He knows I'm trying to help him and happy feelings flood through my veins while I'm extracting blood from his. The gentle noises and openly curious facial expressions of alpacas or llamas lift the spirits and could warm even the coldest of hearts. A baby donkey nuzzles its keeper, or the lucky vet who happens to arrive to check its health soon after it has been born. Joy spreads infectiously to everyone nearby. The unswerving and unconditional happiness of animals is contagious and it makes us humans feel better.

And that is what this book is about. It tells stories of each of the species that I have had the good fortune to look after to try to maintain their happiness. Yes, they are definitely all different, but happy animals are most certainly all alike. And so are we, because happiness is all. I hope you enjoy it.

1. Cows

Cows are curious creatures, gentle and placid. The matriar-chal hierarchy by which the herd is organised lends itself to a calm social situation. Watching cows in a grassy field or straw-filled fold yard, surrounded by their herd-mates, is a relaxing experience. They graze quietly and methodically, gently chewing the cud, or flicking at a fly with their tail. It is no coincidence that the term 'to ruminate' suggests a slow pondering. A calm cow is a peaceful thing.

The first time I had the chance to observe these creatures closely was high up in the Swiss Alps, during the summer of 1993, exactly halfway through studying my veterinary degree at university. I was camping with some friends in a beautiful alpine meadow, which we used as a base for climbing the huge moun-tains nearby – the Täschhorn, Weisshorn, Monte Rosa and Matterhorn. The scene could have been straight from an episode of *Heidi* – the grass was scattered with hundreds of jewel-like flowers and each of the brown and white cows had a huge, clanking bell round its neck. The continuous low clopping of the bells alerted the herdsman to the location of the cows so they didn't get lost. It also alerted the four young climbers from Yorkshire to their proximity. Over the few weeks that we were camping in their meadow, we got to know the cows quite well. In fact, we practically became a part of their herd. It turned out that they were just as interested in us as we were in them, and they would often stick their heads into the unzipped mouths of our tents to wake us up on a morning or just to investigate.

While I loved the herd of which we had become a part, Dave, one of my climbing-mates, developed a correspondingly vigorous hatred of the creatures, quickly dubbing them 'cow bastards'. There was some justification for this hatred, because their behaviour could sometimes be irksome. On one occasion, they ate his entire supply of porridge oats, so breakfasts became a shadow of their former selves. On another, with very different consequences, they ate his spare underpants. The climbers and the cows eventually managed a peaceful coexistence, once Dave had managed to rig up a defence system of climbing rope around the camp. The cattle thought it was an electric fence and from then on kept their distance. What remained of our breakfast ingredients was safe and so were our remaining pants. Human ingenuity had saved the day.

Since those halcyon alpine days and qualifying as a fully fledged vet, I have obviously become more closely connected with cows. I have seen them practically every day and had my hands and arms in almost every part of their capacious anatomy. I've studied them when healthy and when sick, I've removed nails from their rumens, rubber rings from their feet, and tumours from their teats and even (on a few occasions) their diseased eyeballs. I've lost count of the number of calves I have delivered, on windswept moors and in freezing barns, with drizzle spraying between the gaps in the Yorkshire boarding of the cowshed. I've also lost count of the number of shirts I've ruined with bloody obstetrical fluids spilling down the front, or whose rolled-up sleeves have taken on an indelible brownish-green stain after a day of arm-numbing pregnancy testing. I can recollect, in clear detail, the well-aimed kicks – from not-so-benign bovines – and exactly which part of my anatomy they connected with. While I am not, technically, a veterinary expert on cows, I am (or at least have been) a cow-vet. I reflect back on those huge and gentle, doe-eyed Swiss brown cows, because they were the start of a long and intimate relationship with this amazing species.

Nowadays though, in this climate of global warming, cows often get a bad press. It is a complex situation and one that is way beyond the scope of this book. I am not an atmospheric chemist (though I have two good friends who are, and it is a topic that frequently crops up after dinner or over a glass of wine), nor am I a ruminant nutritionist. I do know that cows produce methane during the process of rumination. Methane is a potent greenhouse gas, much more potent than carbon dioxide. However, as every chemistry student knows, methane is very reactive and therefore lasts in the atmosphere for a relatively short period of time. This is in contrast with carbon dioxide, which – unless it happens to come into contact with a molecule of chlorophyll, a molecule of water and a photon of light, whereupon it is turned into part of a plant – hangs around for ages and is a major player in the greenhouse effect, trapping heat in the atmosphere and thereby causing the Earth to warm. Too many greenhouse gases resulting in too much warmth is an inescapable truism. The part played by cows in this is less clear, but nevertheless they are having a bad time of it and could do with a new team of publicists. Like I say, it is complicated.

What is also complicated is getting any nutritional benefit

from grass. Plant cell walls are made of cellulose, which cannot be digested by mammals. Cows and other ruminants manage not just to survive, but to thrive on this basic diet by making use of a whole smorgasbord of symbiotic bugs to do the job that the mammalian digestive system cannot, thereby releasing all the nutrients the grass has to offer. If you live on grass and don't have a rumen – if you're a horse or a rabbit, for example – your intestines have to be enormously long to digest the cellulose and those vital microbes are right at the end (which is why rabbits pass all their food through their digestive system twice). Cows use their rumen for this job. It is a huge vat of fermenting herbage. The grass is chewed to break the cell walls, swallowed, churned in the rumen so the microbes can do their work, then brought back up into the mouth and partly digested for a second chew. Nothing is rushed if you're a cow and it is this melancholic ruminating that makes a cow so endearing, whether she's digesting hay, grass, silage or underpants.

In the words of an old farmer whom I have known for many years: 'You can't beat a good old cow!'

And even though they breathe out methane and eat underpants, she's not far wrong!

Slow Fever and a Journey in the Fog

The miserable November weather was gnawing away at my spirit but, despite the cold and damp, I enjoyed the visit to see Mr Newbold at Apple Tree Farm. The farmer always made me smile, with his funny stories and his slightly alternative view of the farming world. One day, for example, while we were discussing the perilous financial situation of the dairy industry, he commented: 'It's the big boys in this business that I feel sorry for; all that cost. It must be hard to make ends meet.' In a time when it was *only* possible to make a living milking cows by applying the of economies of scale, he had delightfully missed the point.

Mr Newbold's small farm was situated about half a mile from the practice. It was not *the* closest to the practice – that privilege belonged to the farm just over the road, where it was almost quicker to walk there than to drive, provided you could stuff your pockets with everything you might need. But it only took a couple of minutes to get to Apple Tree Farm, where Mr Newbold kept a handful of old-fashioned, black-and-white dairy cows, all with horns, fastened up side by side in a byre, where they would munch on hay throughout the long winter months. In summer, they grazed in a small paddock next to the main road into Thirsk. Apple trees and a hawthorn hedge lined the paddock and, as I drove to work each morning, I could catch glimpses of the cows and heifers through the gaps in the trees and the holes in the hedge. I always tried to see what they were up to because, to Mr Newbold, the behaviour of his cows was an accurate predictor of what the weather might have in store. Whether his cows were standing up or lying down and in which direction their bodies were pointing was, in his opinion, as good as the Met Office for a weather forecast. He used other natural clues too, to prognosticate about the harshness of the winter ahead, the persistence of the latest wet period or even the conditions five miles away, at the top of Sutton Bank. Elevated three hundred metres above the Vale of York where Mr Newbold's farm was situated, it could be a completely different world at the top of Sutton Bank. There could be snow when there was rain in Thirsk; there could be fog when it was simply cloudy and overcast below; and, on the odd occasion, when there was thick fog lingering along the Vale, a drive up the steep road could bring you popping out above the clouds, just like a ride in an aeroplane!

Even when Mr Newbold called the vet for help, he always had his own diagnosis. His bovine diagnosis was always followed by a meteorological prediction about how the weather would unfold during the week. Rumour had it that Mr Newbold learnt his tricks from Thirsk's famous amateur weather forecaster, Bill Foggitt.

Bill was born in Thirsk in 1913, the latest in a long line of local weather forecasters. He had lived not far away from Apple Tree Farm – hence the assumption that this was where he'd acquired his skills. His family had run a chemist's shop in the marketplace for many generations. In 1771 the area was hit by a great flood, during which part of North Yorkshire's most northerly town, Yarm, was washed away by the swollen River Tees. Bill's ancestors were both horrified and intrigued and began to make meticulous observations of anything from the unseasonal arrival of a flock of waxwings, or the erratic behaviour of sheep, to the habits of moles, to try to find patterns that might allow them to predict and prepare for future extreme events. The rate of desiccation or otherwise of certain types of seaweed was a favourite tool. This knowledge and insight was passed down through the generations, conferring upon the family the status of some sort of Yorkshire soothsayer, but without the sacrifice or the entrails.

I'm sure Mr Newbold had developed and built upon the Foggitt theories, adding cows to the formulary and working on refining and improving the accuracy. I was certain that my visit to see his poorly cow on this November afternoon would also afford me a weather forecast.

'Ah! Now then, thanks for coming,' he bellowed, even though he was standing right next to the open window of the driver's-side door of my car as I pulled up in the yard. He was always anxious to crack on, ready and waiting when the vet arrived. For this, I am always grateful. One of the deep frustrations of being a large animal vet is when, on a tight schedule, you get to a farm to find no sign of the farmer or the patient and have to set about searching sheds and outbuildings for one, the other or both.

'I have a cow with slow fever,' Mr Newbold went on, as I climbed out of the car. 'It is slow fever, I know that, because I can smell it,' he added with certainty, before marching off in the direction of his cowshed. He wasn't a young man, but he retained a youthful supply of energy and always seemed to be starting one job before he'd finished the last.

There was a reasonable chance he was right with his diagnosis. That it is possible to detect slow fever in a cow by smell does have a basis in fact – probably more so than using the flowering of coltsfoot to predict the weather. Slow fever, contrary to the suggestion in its name, does not mean the herd ambles around at half speed. It is a metabolic disorder that can affect recently calved cows. It is characterised by an energy deficiency, triggered by the sudden demand for an udder full of lactose-rich milk. To make milk, glucose is taken from the blood and other body tissues and, if sufficient food is not eaten to replace this crucial energy source, the blood glucose levels plummet.

There are reasons why a cow might not eat sufficient food: she might be poorly after calving and therefore not feel like eating; she could be too fat, so that her appetite is insufficient; or she might not have access to enough food. In each of these cases, the body tries to use its supplies of body fat to correct the energy gap. This works quite well for a short time, but the prolonged metabolism of body fat leads to a build-up of ketones in the blood and this causes something called ketosis. The presence of ketones in the bloodstream has a suppressive effect on the appetite, exacerbating the problem further and creating a vicious circle of energy depletion and ever-increasing levels of ketones. Slow fever's proper name is acetonaemia, which describes this unhealthy build-up of ketones in the blood. Some people can smell ketones on a cow's breath – they have the aroma of pear drops – and this makes a diagnosis simple. Apparently this ability is a genetic trait, impossible to learn; you can either smell the ketones or you can't. But, while being able to make a diagnosis by smell is useful, there is still the issue of finding a *reason* for the reduced appetite, and treating the signs. That is where the vet comes in, and where a stethoscope, thermometer, rectal glove and so on come into play.

I put on my wellies and grabbed each of these bits of kit, along with my little pot of magic diagnostic powder, and followed Mr Newbold into the cowshed.

He was already in position, hand on the withers of his cow, inhaling her pear-scented breath by the lungful.

'Yep, it's definitely slow fever! Her milk's dropped and look, smell her!' he instructed, pushing the cow's mouth towards me. I smiled slightly at the idea of looking at a smell. There was always something to amuse me on a visit to Apple Tree Farm. I enjoy a pear drop and I can fully appreciate the chemistry-lab aroma, but I have never been convinced I can actually make a diagnosis of acetonaemia with my nose. (There is a renowned cattle veterinary book that contains the classic line 'some prac-titioners can *smell* salmonellosis', as if to add weight to the power of the nose when it comes to making a thorough clinical exam-ination.) This was where my magic powder came in. Of course, it wasn't actually magic, but the result of mixing it with the milk or urine of a ketotic cow had a magical effect on many a scep-tical farmer. In my opinion, it is an underused technique; and the younger generation of vets seem completely unaware of its existence. Presumably the veterinary specialists advise blood sampling to get a full profile of the energy status. This is just as helpful but more time-consuming and more costly. My powder is called Rothera's reagent and provides an immediate diagnosis, as the cream-coloured powder turns a regal purple in the pres-ence of ketones. I always use it when I see a cow that has stopped eating.

Usually an examination follows a prescribed pattern. In a dog, I usually start at the head and work backward, culminating in the taking of the temperature. With a lame leg, I start at the bottom, wiggling each toe, squeezing each pad and examining each interdigital space in turn. Working up the leg, I manipulate each joint and check along the limb until I've found the source of pain: dogs can't say 'It hurts just here,' so vets need to rely on eliciting some sort of reaction. When the dog winces, then I know for certain where it hurts.

But with cows, my examination varies depending on which bit is the most likely to be causing the problem and which bits are the most easily accessible. In this case, the cows were all lined up, fastened, in an old-fashioned byre, waiting to be milked. Several rear ends were facing me, so it was easiest to do all the stuff at the back end first – temperature measurement and then internal examination. Next came the udder, to feel its consistency, to check for mastitis and to take a sample of milk to mix with the Rothera's reagent. Sure enough, just as we'd both expected, the off-white powder in its little pot turned first pink, then deep purple, confirming to diagnosis of acetonaemia.

'Look at that!' I called to Mr Newbold, holding the purple vial high in the air. Even though I've done this test many times, I'm always impressed by a chemical reaction that elicits such a dramatic colour change. I will always be a chemist at heart!

The rest of my examination did not uncover any other health issues, so it was a simple fix. Steroids work brilliantly for slow fever, almost as magically as the Rothera's powder does to provide a diagnosis. In severe cases, where the cow has become delirious as a result of the high level of ketones in the blood (nervous acetonaemia), the animal will go bonkers, charging around wildly and manically licking anything in front of them, especially metal bars. Their ears flick relentlessly as if they are picking up strange sounds or voices in their heads, and their eyeballs bulge with surprise and confusion. These cases need more vigorous treatment. Intravenous glucose injections and oral supplementation work well, just as jelly babies help a hypoglycaemic diabetic patient.

Mr Newbold's cow was not that bad. He'd spotted it early. I was as certain that my treatment would be effective as we both were about the diagnosis. Mr Newbold held the sweet-smelling cow by her head so I could perform an intravenous injection. The jugular vein of a cow is large and prominent, and it is a straightforward job to identify the target and inject the medicine. Even if it is not possible to see the vein, by tapping the area with the middle finger you can locate it, as it vibrates, while placing the hand not holding the syringe on the side of the neck, pressing across the vein, to make the jugular, as big as a hosepipe, bulge. The partial and temporary obstruction to blood flow in the vein makes it distend and its feeling is unmistakable. You can literally feel the fluidity of the blood, standing in a column an inch and a half across. The needle went in, spilling crimson venous blood all over my fingers. It is always messy, but I prefer to insert the needle before it is attached to the syringe. It is a safe way to ensure that the injection goes into exactly the right place.

Once I was all done, I rinsed my bloody hands and washed my wellies. Mr Newbold and I chatted for a while, as we always did after treating a patient, and he showed me some of his cattle, like a proud parent at sports day or after receiving a glowing school report. He introduced each one – 'look at this for a calf!' – before giving me all the details of its delivery, the age of its mum along with any relevant (or irrelevant) facts about her health and history. Even though his herd was small, this seemed to take for ever, so I was glad when my phone rang. It was the practice, sending me off on another call. I nodded and made some notes on the back of my hand about where it was and the nature of the problem. The farm was one I hadn't been to before. It was called Dry Rigg Farm and it was up at the top of Sutton Bank. I scribbled directions, which I knew would not be adequate.

Apparently, the farm was deep inside a thick forest. It sounded as if I would be looking for Hansel and Gretel's cottage and I'd need to lay a trail of crumbs to avoid being lost for ever. The instructions were vague. I was to turn left off the so-called main road (it was anything but main) to Sproxton, onto a forest track, then bear right at the second fork in the track, after which time it became a bit rough, apparently. I had to look out for a small, wooden signpost with the words Dry Rigg inscribed. I didn't fancy my chances, especially as it was already foggy and would be getting dark soon.

Mr Newbold asked, with genuine interest, what I had to do next.

'It's a calf that's sick,' I explained. 'But it's at the top of Sutton Bank, in the middle of the forest.'

'Ah! That'll be pneumonia, that will,' he prognosticated. 'A cold and damp evening like this, all the wetness and chill in the air. As sure as eggs are eggs that calf will have pneumonia.'

Pneumonia is a common ailment for cattle, especially in the dank days of November when the chill and damp air allows a dangerous concoction of viruses, bacteria and other microbes to thrive. We always treat these cases with utmost urgency, because the lung damage can be so sudden and so severe that an animal can deteriorate rapidly and die within a day. Mr Newbold was probably right, but I smiled at the certainty of his diagnosis, made without his trusty nose and without even laying eyes on the little calf.

'And it'll be a bad place to be,' he added, without even turning to his cows for a prediction. 'It's going to be thick fog up there on a night like this. It'll be pitch black and you'll not be able to see your hand in front of your face. It's sure to be a proper pea-souper!'

He was sure to be right on this point, too. It didn't take a master weather forecaster to tell me that; I'd spent enough time at the top of Sutton Bank, after dark and in the grim depths of winter, to know that I would be in for a long and slow journey, nothing like the three-minute trip I'd just done, with a simple treatment and a guaranteed cure. I braced myself for yet another challenge.

Cast Your Bread

It was a busy day. The morning had been jam-packed with small animal consultations – a cat with a sore eye, a couple of limping dogs, post-op checks, inflamed ears and dodgy bowels. The list was already full, but extras kept appearing. Given my increasing tendency to chat at length to clients, sometimes about their pets but often about something completely different, I was running late, overstretched and slightly stressed. My final patients came in all together: a family of rabbits, all in need of vaccination. Their owners had rescued a number rabbits over recent months, out of kindness and an interest in this curious species. But a shortage of hutch space for the newly rescued rabbits, along with the problems for a rabbit novice inherent with sexing youngsters, had resulted in a population explosion in an otherwise tranquil garden in North Yorkshire. It was just five to vaccinate this time – a lot of rabbits to see at once, but fewer than at their previous visit. One of them was a baby giant rabbit, whose ears were bigger than his body.

At last the waiting room was empty. I wiped the table and slumped into a chair to write up my notes. Should I grab a coffee or get some food? It was a perennial question for a busy vet, yet another lunchtime had been swallowed up by the urgent needs of my patients.

In the end, it was neither. The boss was playing golf, we had an influx of new clients, all of whom, apparently, needed their animals seeing immediately, and one vet was on a well-earned half-day, so the afternoon looked as if it was going to be as busy as the morning. But it was full of a different kind of work, out and about, in the fields and on the farms of North Yorkshire. It was lucky that a change is (apparently) as good as a rest. I headed straight out to see Mr Morris and his cow.

The message in the daybook told some of the story. Mr Morris had a cow down, recumbent and unable to stand. Downer cows such as this could be challenging to deal with, in part because there are several conditions all of which might result in the same problem for the cow. When I was a young, recently qualified vet, I would spend the drive to the farm running through in my mind all the possible diagnoses and the ways of distinguishing one from another; could it be one of the many mineral deficiencies that cows are prone to? Would I need to take some blood to check these levels? It could be toxaemia from an infection in the udder or uterus, in which case I would need antibiotics and anti-inflammatories rather than big bottles of mineral solution; maybe it was something physical – a damaged pelvis as a result of a difficult calving, or maybe just impingement on a nerve, giving a bad case of sciatica – a common sequel to a tricky delivery. Nowadays, this list is thoroughly ingrained in my subconscious, and I just wait to see what I find when I get there.

Mr Morris was waiting anxiously in the yard when I arrived. His farm, perched high on the hill, was straight out of a James Herriot book, with ancient, sagging gates patched up with baler twine and rustic wooden feed troughs spilling over with hay and silage. He ushered me into the building where my patient was lying, not looking particularly poorly but clearly making no attempt to get to her feet.

I set about my examination, as I had done so many times before. The first step was to take the animal's temperature, so I rummaged in my box for a thermometer.

'Is that a glass thermometer?' the elderly farmer asked, obviously delighted by this equally old piece of equipment. Alongside his ancient buildings, the glass and mercury device was not out of place.

'It is.' I nodded. 'You don't see many around these days.'

'I can't get used to these modern, beeping ones,' Mr Morris complained. 'I can't read 'em. They never seem to get the right temperature and then they run out of batteries.'

I withdrew the slim glass instrument from the cow's rectum, and he came round to peer at it. He was more animated than I'd ever seen him, and there was real envy in his eyes.

'Where do you get them from?' he asked longingly.

'Well, you can't buy them any more,' I explained, 'but I have a secret stash of a few that were given to me by a retired nurse. Each one comes with its own little metal case. They are really nice things and just as accurate as the modern ones.'

As I worked my way through the examination, listening to the stomach and the lungs, checking the udder, manipulating the limbs and performing an internal examination, I could see Mr Morris out of the corner of my eye. Normally, the farmer watches closely, anxiously waiting to hear the verdict on his animal. But I could tell Mr Morris was more interested in the ancient (but still very accurate) thermometer, which I had now replaced carefully in its metal case.

I came to a diagnosis of post-partum obturator neuritis, which is inflammation of one of the nerves that has been squashed by the calf squeezing through the pelvic canal. These cases usually respond quite well to injections of anti-inflammatories, so I went back to the car to make up a syringe for injection. While I was there, I had another idea. I checked my supply of thermometers. These slivers of glass and mercury are ephemeral things, prone to immediate breakage if they come into contact with anything hard. Even if they don't come into contact with anything hard they tend to vanish. Once at vet school, a friend was taking the temperature of a young foal that was suffering from a joint infection. The foal contracted his anus at exactly the wrong moment and the thermometer disappeared, as did the foal, careering off across the paddock. We spent hours searching through the grass and scrutinising foal-sized faeces in the hope of finding the missing object. It never reappeared.

Anyway, I returned to the cow to give the all-important injection. Then, I reached into my pocket and presented Mr Morris with my spare metal-case-clad, glass-and-mercury thermometer.

'And this is for you,' I said. 'Don't lose it and don't drop it. As you know, you can't get them any more.'

The effect on the farmer was more dramatic than the effect of my treatment on the cow. A huge beam spread across his wrinkled face. I have rarely seen a farmer so happy.

As I drove off I caught a glimpse of Mr Morris in my rear-view mirror. He was still lovingly clutching his gift. I was glad to have been able to cheer him up. As my mum used to say, 'It's nice to be important, but it's more important to be nice.'

The day continued in its busy vein and it wasn't long before I was out on the road again. Another cow – this one struggling to calve – and another old, traditional Yorkshire farmer.

I arrived to see the Friesian already standing in the cattle crush, with the enormous, crossed-over feet of a huge calf protruding. It didn't need a vet to diagnose that this calf was way too big to be born naturally and would need a Caesarean section.

Everything went super-smoothly. The patient was impeccably behaved and I had lots of helpers – it was a large family and brothers, cousins and uncles were all on hand. Some were taking photographs, while others prepared syringes for me, filled buckets with warm water or fetched and carried. I also had a table on which to place all my equipment, so it was altogether a perfect set-up and the mood was upbeat. I soon had the calf out. It was enormous but fit and healthy. Two of the three brothers lifted it into a wheelbarrow to move it onto to a safe and clean straw bed, while I sutured everything back together.

'Would yer look at that!' exclaimed Derek, the other brother. 'T'old girl is actually chewing her cud, right while yer stitching her back together! Chewing her cud – you can't get a more contented cow than that!'

I was finished before long and cleaned off and packed up, but before I returned to my car Derek said, 'Julian, you've done a fantastic job this evening. We were worried, but it was the best thing to do. So, 'ave some eggs and these little onions. As a bit of a thank-you like!'

He held out a tray of thirty eggs and four of the biggest onions I'd ever seen, almost as big as footballs!

When I was a young boy, my gran used to give me wise advice. We were close and she was knowledgeable about lots of things. I am glad to have inherited some of her attributes – optimism, enthusiasm, stoicism and just a little bit of her stubbornness. One of her favourite sayings was based on a passage from the New Testament, which advises people to 'cast their bread on the water'. The rest of the story goes on to suggest that by doing this, an act of generosity, rather than just keeping your bread and eating it, you reap greater rewards – happiness, inner contentment and so on. My gran paraphrased this epistle by saying, 'cast your bread on the water and it will come back as ham sandwiches.'

It was good advice. Today I had cast my metaphorical bread in the shape of a vintage thermometer. Instead of coming back as ham sandwiches, it had come back as massive onions. My gran would have been proud.

Maurice and the Milk Fever

It was the Friday night before two weeks off work – a holiday at last, in the peace and sparkling clean air of the French Alps. Anne and the boys were already there, but it was my weekend on call and no one had been able to swap so, instead of Friday night being the start of the holiday, I faced the prospect of two more days at the mercy of my pager. I hoped it would be quiet, because I still had plenty to do – the camper van needed careful packing for the long journey and it wouldn't do it on its own! But my hopes were dashed by a call late in the evening. It had been a pleasant day and it was still warm and light. Only just light – dusk was fast approaching as I arrived at the farm to meet Maurice, the farmer – the epitome of Yorkshire tradition – waiting at the rickety gate, leaning on his pickup.

'Have we got problems?' I asked. I was aware from the message on my beeper that there was a cow struggling and I knew he'd requested an urgent visit, but the details were sketchy.

'Yes, we have,' he muttered gruffly. 'It's a cow. She completely conked out, like. She's not even here, she's away in a field so you'll have to follow me.'

He hopped into his vehicle, switched on the lights and disappeared down the track. I followed, as swiftly as was safe and as my recently acquired extra speeding points would allow. I could see Maurice's rear lights disappearing into the distance ahead of me, but luckily this was one of the uber-straight roads along which hundreds of Roman soldiers would have marched as they conquered the north of Britain, about two thousand years ago. I kept the vehicle in sight, until it turned down a narrow and by now quite dark lane. Luckily Maurice paused to wait for me, because what followed was a series of lefts and rights into what seemed like absolutely nowhere. Already I was beginning to worry about my return journey once I had fixed the 'conked-out' cow, and I started to make mental notes of trees and corners and gates so that I could retrace my steps.

Eventually Maurice pulled over onto a verge and came round to talk to me, through my open window.

'She's in there, like,' he said, nodding towards a wooden, five-bar gate that had seen better days. It was not so much a gate as a collection of planks of wood connected together by bits of baler twine. But this was not the next problem.

'It's a field of rigs and furrows, so you might struggle in your car. Do you want to have a lift, bring your stuff with you, like? She's down – completely conked out,' he reiterated, before continuing, 'I think it might be magnesium deficiency. Or calcium. Or mastitis. She just calved the other day, yer see.'

I asked a few more questions, trying to glean enough information to give me an idea of why she might have 'conked out'.

'She looked a bit wobbly at six, when I came to check 'em,' Maurice explained, 'so I went to fetch some gates to make a pen. And then I'd made a pen but when I came back she'd gone flat out and couldn't get up, like. And that's when I thought I'd call you. I thought she might be dead by morning, otherwise.'

This gave me a clear image of the cow and her problem, and I gathered what I'd need – calcium solution, magnesium solution, an orange tube called a flutter valve to run the appropriate solution into the cow's vein, a halter to catch her with and, of course, some wide-bore needles so the liquid would run in smoothly. I grabbed a few in case any got lost in the dark, or bent – I didn't want to have to come back to my car. There is nothing worse, in the middle of a field in the dark, than the mineral solution running in too slowly because the needle has blocked or is too narrow. I had some new ones with clear plastic ends and a green case that would be ideal. They had superseded the old style fourteen-gauge needles, which came in an orange needle case. I stuffed three into my pocket and jumped into the pickup alongside Maurice, who set off across the bumpy and rutted field. Even though my own Subaru was a 4x4 and adept off-road, the tussocky nature of the grass and the large furrows and 'rigs' (ridges) would have risked the health of my exhaust pipe. The other cows in the field would present a further hazard, as they would be sure to come over to investigate the excitement. I'd had many near misses with wing mirrors in the past and, at the very least, the licking tongues of curious cows leave a wind-screen smeared with tenacious gloop. I was happy to leave my car outside the gate. After all, I had everything I would need.

We made slow progress through the lumpy field, but eventually we spotted the patient lying comfortably amongst her friends, who were all standing up. From a distance, in the headlights of Maurice's vehicle and surrounded by her herd-mates, she didn't look too bad.

'Oh, heck. Don't say she's better already!' exclaimed Maurice.

It seemed that she did not look as bad now as she had an

hour earlier (she had, after all, been completely conked out), but as I got out of the passenger seat and went to investigate, the poor cow struggled to her feet and wobbled and tottered her way off into the darkness, looking extremely poorly. With the help of Maurice's headlights and my trusty head-torch, I managed to get the halter round her head before she disappeared into the night. That was the first hurdle negotiated. The burst of effort had been too much for the stricken animal and she flopped to the ground. Maurice leant on her neck so she wouldn't move. I fitted the bottle of mineral mixture onto my flutter valve. The mixture contained all the important things for a cow like this: calcium, magnesium, phosphate and glucose. A deficiency in the blood levels of any or all of these things is quite common in cows shortly after they've given birth. The sudden demand for milk in the udder to feed the newborn calf puts an enormous strain on the system. The result is a wobbly cow, or worse one that cannot stand up.

Now, all I needed to do was attach the orange tube to a needle placed in the jugular vein. I pulled one of my needles from my pocket and snapped off the case. What appeared from within made my heart sink. It was a slender nineteen-gauge needle, and not the fourteen-gauge one I'd expected. Fourteen-gauge needles are wide and suitable for administering an injection fast into a large vein. Nineteen-gauge ones are narrow and only suitable for injecting small volumes from a small syringe. I cursed under my breath, both at myself for not double-checking my equipment, and at whichever marketing department had thought it would be a good idea to change the packaging of the needles. They clearly had not tried finding kit in a hurry in the dark. I was faced with two options – go back to the car for the bigger needles, or use the ones I had, which would mean the liquid trickling in very slowly, over about ten or fifteen minutes per bottle, rather than quickly over about two. It was a long way back to the car and we had already caught the cow. It seemed silly to retrace our bumpy journey. Besides, it was a warm evening and standing in a dark field, surrounded by curious cows, might even be seen by some as a form of meditative retreat. I'd heard stories of people doing yoga with goats – maybe 'tantric cow infusions' would catch on as a way of unwinding on a Friday night?

By the look of the cow, she was going to need three bottles of calcium, which would take at least half an hour, but I decided to take the slow option. It wouldn't do any harm. It might even do me good – it was being in a rush that had caused the problem in the first place. 'Blooming newfangled packaging!', I thought to myself.

Slow as the progress was, it was still progress. The cow was on her side, as Maurice had pinned her down and was keeping her halter tight, while the telltale burping that started shortly after the mineral mix began to trickle into her blood was a sure sign that her low calcium levels were rising. Calcium is crucial for muscle contraction, and some of the weakness associated with the condition of milk fever is quickly corrected as the levels revert to normal.* The burping is the result of the rumen kicking back into life. This means that, even without the benefit of a blood sample, a clinician can easily tell if the bovine patient is responding to treatment.

But as the cow's problems started to resolve, another problem

---

* Cows can succumb to all manner of conditions, many described as 'fever'. Some are apt – slow fever makes a cow slow; milk fever develops after a cow has come to her milk; shipping fever develops after a bovine has moved from one farm to another; red water fever leads to blood-tinged urine. Some have less obvious names, such as fog fever, triggered by eating the wrong sort of grass rather than anything to do with misty pastures.

developed. Maurice had put two large bags of tasty cow-cake in the back of his pickup, to tempt the herd into his recently constructed pen. The animals had discovered this and were trying to climb into the back of the vehicle to eat it.

'Here, hold this,' he said, giving me the halter rope to hold with my free hand, while in the other one I held the calcium bottle as high as I could to get it to run in more quickly, 'They're all eating my food and I'm worried about my truck.'

As Maurice slackened his hold on her, the cow spotted her chance to escape and leapt to her feet. The needle came out of her vein, I lost control of the halter and the cow, still wobbly, careered off across the field like a drunk at a party. Luckily, because she was still confused, Maurice quite quickly managed to recapture her and fasten the rope to the tow-bracket of the pickup. Normal service was resumed and I reached for a second bottle.

'That was a near miss,' I said, as I lifted my head-torch to check his wing mirrors. They were all intact.

'Once I was doing this with a vet,' recalled the farmer, 'and the cow stood up, ran off and ran straight into the vet's car! She ended up sitting on the bonnet!'

I'd seen similar things happen before. At the very start of my veterinary career, I worked in the far north of Scotland. During that halcyon summer I treated cows with almost every condition imaginable, including many cases of milk fever (calcium deficiency) and grass staggers (magnesium deficiency). Most of them were out in fields, so the first problem was coping with the midges; the second was retrieving a lost halter when, the minute she felt even slightly better, the wild beast jumped to her feet and crazily charged off over the horizon. I lost a lot of halters that summer!

The second bottle trickled into the cow even more slowly than the first. I'd opted to use a double-strength bottle of 40 per cent solution this time. It must have been more thick and syrupy

– my index and middle fingers had actually stuck together because of the extra sugar in the second bottle. It was a bit like injecting treacle.

But then another problem presented itself.

'I'm just a bit worried about my battery,' Maurice admitted. 'I'll hold your bottle if you can go and switch off the headlights. If the battery runs out we really are stuck.'

So, we swapped roles again and I clambered into the driver's side of the vehicle to find the light switch. Certainly, the lights had dimmed considerably. This was another problem I had experienced before, while calving a cow in a dark field. I was smugly enjoying the most brightly illuminated nocturnal calving ever until the moment I tried to drive off, and found I had a completely dead car! This would be a major headache tonight in this rutted field, surrounded by cows, in the pitch black save for the cone of light from my head-torch – I dared not contemplate its battery life at this point.

Without the headlights it was very dark and the patient, feeling stronger by the minute, was making more and more frequent attempts to escape. With the second bottle nearly empty, a final swing of her back end signified that she had had enough – both literally and figuratively. She had had sufficient calcium solution and she was fed up with being restrained. I pulled out the needle and wiped my sticky hands on the damp, dewy grass. Maurice, meanwhile, fumbled to unfasten the halter, which by now had become tightly wrapped around the tow-bracket of his vehicle.

Eventually, the cow was free and my hands were marginally less sticky. We watched her trot off into the night, looking for her calf. It hadn't been the most straightforward of evenings, but at least she was over the worst of it. We climbed into the truck and looked at each other anxiously as Maurice turned the key. A flicker of life, but no engine noise. He tried again. This time, to our relief, the rusty pickup lurched into some sort of life and we set off to make the slow, bumpy journey back to where I'd left my car. An awful thought came to me as we trundled across the rutted fields – had I switched off my own car headlights?

The rest of the weekend progressed in a similar vein, so to speak. A young feral cat, who had made herself a new home with a local family, had started giving birth. The first kitten was born at 9 p.m., but no more had appeared and by three in the morning the adopted owners were worried. So, there was not much sleep during the small hours. I'd just got back into bed when the phone rang again. This time, it was a dairy cow that had tried to jump a barbed wire fence. The result was a large wound under her tummy. She was at one of our furthest farms and, according to the farmer, blood was spurting everywhere, so there was no time even for a cup of coffee before heading out to start Saturday morning. The camper van was no closer to being packed, although the holiday was approaching fast. I couldn't wait. It would be a relaxing and a much-needed break – at least it would once the seventeen-hour drive had been completed. I hoped it wouldn't be me that conked out before I got there!

Death at Embleton's

To paraphrase Robbie Burns, 'The best laid plans of mice and men often go awry'. It's a phrase that can be applied to most days as a veterinary surgeon in mixed practice. Obviously, mice don't make very many plans, let alone ones that have been laid well, but certainly the best-laid plans of vets seem to be thwarted fairly regularly. And so it was on this particular morning.

My best-laid plan was to visit an elderly gentleman and his young dog. I'd operated on the dog a couple of weeks before and it was time for his sutures to be removed. The gentleman had been in hospital too, so I had arranged to call in to save him struggling to the surgery. He lived close to the practice so I planned to go on my way into work, before the vagaries of the day and its emergencies presented themselves. All I needed to do was set off from home ten minutes earlier than usual. It would be a good use of time. Or so I thought.

But, just as I set off, my mobile phone rang. It was my boss with another call for me.

'Julian. Alan here,' came the voice from the car speakers.

'Can you call and see Mr Embleton on your way?' he continued, 'It's quite urgent and I have to go to do a whole load of pregnancy scans over near Nidderdale. It's fixed up for nine and I can't be late. He's worried about this cow – she's about a week off calving and is down. It doesn't sound good. You know what he's like, he only wants you or me to go.'

'Yep, that's fine,' I replied, 'I was on my way to see Henry the German Shepherd to take out his sutures – his owner can't leave the house 'cos he's just had an operation too – but I expect that can wait. I don't have his number, but if someone at the practice could call him to let him know I'll be late, that would be good.'

Alan agreed to get the message to Henry's owner while I worked out the best way of getting to Mr Embleton's farm. I had been a couple of times before but, on both occasions, I had gone directly from the practice. This time I would have to take the back roads, as I was approaching from a different direction. By the sounds of it, time was very much of the essence. As I wound my way along the twisting lanes of North Yorkshire, some of which I hadn't been along before, I racked my brains for a reason that Mr Embleton's cow might be down before calving. He had a decent-sized dairy herd, over a hundred cows, and it was pretty well run, although quite old-fashioned and traditional. His cows enjoyed sunshine on their backs and grass in their bellies during the summer months, and were generally healthy and happy. For a cow to be recumbent and very poorly *before* she had calved signified something very seriously wrong. The common complaints affecting dairy cows usually develop after calving – milk fever, mastitis, nerve damage from a difficult calving, metritis, displaced stomach or slow fever (ketosis), for example.

When examining a sick cow, the first thing to do is to ask the farmer when she calved. The second thing is to ask if she ate her breakfast and the third thing is to ask how much milk she gave that morning. Armed with these three bits of information, a veterinary surgeon already has some important clues, even before reaching for a stethoscope or inserting a thermometer. But all these questions relate to a cow that has already calved. In truth, there were not many illnesses that would make a dry cow (one who hasn't yet calved) so sick that she couldn't rise. Equally, there were very few conditions that would make Mr Embleton so worried that he would call a vet out with such urgency.

It wasn't just that he was tight with his money, or no more so than many Yorkshire farmers. He never seemed to have much faith in our ability to cure his cows. He would try all his own remedies first before going to the expense of calling a vet. It is a self-fulfilling prophesy that I have seen many times before: 'I'll try not to get the vet out; it'll save me a few bob,' is the common thought process. By the time the vet is finally called, after the cow, sheep or pig has failed to respond to the full repertoire of home treatments, it has often deteriorated to a point that there is no hope of a cure. The despondent vet injects several syringes full of drugs in the hope that at least one of them will help. The result is an expensive bill (we used three syringes, you see) and an animal that doesn't respond to treatment. It confirms what the farmer thought in the first place – 'what a waste of time calling that vet out. I'll not waste me money next time!' And the cycle continues.

But this was not the case today. The patient had been normal the previous evening (apparently) but, overnight, had become extremely ill. I rushed as much as the roads would allow, cautiously making my way up a lane carrying a warning sign about a severe gradient and unsuitability for coaches. It was steep, winding and narrow, with overhanging bracken and brambles on both sides making the lane narrower now, in summer, than they were in winter, but at least there was no ice to contend with. Despite the urgency of the call, I couldn't help but enjoy the drive. With the sun burning off the early-morning mist, flocks of lapwings with their haphazard flight and their strange peeping noise and little rabbits scurrying in front of the car to squeeze under gates into the dew-covered fields beyond, it was not a bad journey to work.

Finally, down another steep hill, across a ford and then up another steep climb, and I arrived at Mr Embleton's farm. He was there, waiting at the gate, waving me to another entrance.

'Go in the next one,' he called. 'She's out in the field.'

I followed his directions round a sharp bend and up another track into the yard. I drove in slowly – the surface was uneven and full of potholes and when I pulled up in approximately the right place, the hobbling and slightly stooped farmer had beaten me to it. He was pointing at a wooden and five-bar gate, optimistically held together with faded orange baler twine and reclining at a gentle angle.

'Can I drive into the field?' I asked. I love to drive into a field, partly because it makes it easier to get to all my equipment without walking back and forth and carrying it all, but mostly because it is a great adventure to negotiate ruts, mud and cows.

'Aye, yer should be alreet,' said the dour old farmer. He was always dour, rarely raising a smile. This is not an uncommon trait in farmers. When I was a veterinary student, encountering farmers for the first time, I used to think their surly, uncommunicative nature was because they were inherently rude, maybe disapproving of a youngster from a town intruding into their own, insular world. I now know that this is not necessarily the case. It is usually because they bear the weight of responsibility for the health and productivity of all their animals, alongside the financial pressures of running a business where the returns are often out of their control. Mr Embleton, for example, could do nothing to control the price he got for the milk he produced. Farmers often work alone, unable to share these pressures with anyone. In the case of dairy farmers in particular, they usually have to get out of bed at half past four in the morning so they are chronically exhausted into the bargain. I could often sympathise.

I edged my way through the lumpy entrance to the field as the stooped farmer held open the gate. He looked even more gloomy than usual today. I hoped I'd be able to make a decent stab at fixing his cow. If not, I feared his mood on this sunny summer's day would slide even further downhill.

'She's not ower good,' he said through the open window of my car as I paused at the gate. 'She was fine yesterday but now she's down, there's some slime at her back end and a bit o' blood. I can't think what's up wi' her. I don't know if there's anything yer can do? And she's gone down rait quick,' he added.

'I came as quickly as I could. Which direction is she?' I asked, scanning the field to try to spy a moribund cow.

He gesticulated over to the right.

Once in the field, I surveyed the scene in more detail. There were several happy-looking heifers, black and white and shiny, near the top of the field. Some were standing eating grass, others lying down and chewing the cud, all equally content. The life of a cow in a sunny field of grass is not a bad one.

One summer, when I was a student, I spent a month working with a dairy herd in Dorset. My job was to supervise the cows as they calved, treat the navel of each calf with iodine soon after it was born and generally help out at this busy time of the year. I actually got paid to stand (or preferably sit on a wall) and watch cows all day.

However, away from the group was the unmistakable form of

my patient. Motionless and flat out, lying on her side, head extended, belly distended. I manoeuvred slowly towards her, Mr Embleton, who had declined a lift, hobbling alongside.

'It doesn't look good, does it?' I said, stating the obvious.

'No. I hope you're not too late,' Mr Embleton replied grimly, also, as it transpired, stating the obvious.

I drew to a halt and got out of the car, prodding the motionless and already rigid cow. I didn't need any more than that to reach my diagnosis.

'I'm afraid I am,' was all I could add, by way of professional assessment, 'I don't think there's anything I can do.' Under the tragic circumstances, it was hard to know what else to say. I braced myself, expecting that this catastrophe would plunge the sombre farmer further into gloom, but the effect was quite the opposite.

'Well, I know you're a good vet, but you're not that good!' he said, laughing heartily at his joke. 'You'll never get her right now, that's for sure! It must have been a twist or sommat. I'm sorry to have wasted your time. It's not a very good start to the day, is it? I'll call the knacker man.'

I was nonplussed – but relieved. Mr Embleton did not seem too upset. He was, as ever, pragmatic through and through. Maybe he was pleased that he hadn't wasted three syringes of expensive drugs on a hopeless case. I started to climb back into my car.

'But I'll tell you what.' A thought had obviously just occurred to him, 'While you're here, you couldn't just have a quick look at a little calf for me could yer? She's just blowin' a bit and I think it *could* be a touch of pneumonia.'

'Of course I can,' I said, smiling inwardly that Mr Embleton had spotted an opportunity to make use of the vet on his farm. Otherwise my visit *would* have been a waste of time – and money. Dour and thrifty. The hallmarks of a typical Yorkshire farmer!

Extirpating Bertha

'I'm worried, Julian,' explained Chris, over the phone. 'It's this eye, it's just not getting any better and, as you know, she's my best cow. It's sore and she's due to give birth any time. And I'm worried. I'm really worried. What can we do?'

I knew Bertha quite well. She was, of course, Chris's favourite cow (although he said that about all of his cows). She was particularly special, though, because she was one of the first Whitebred Shorthorn cows that had arrived at Spring View Farm and was a founder member of this rare-breed herd. Chris was passionate about the breed, partly because of their endearing nature and partly because (as he told me on almost every occasion that we met) the cows were 'rarer than the Giant Panda'. He was doing his best to rectify this. Some months before, I had visited the farm to pregnancy test all his breeding stock, including Bertha. It had been a tense day for Chris, but as we worked our way through the herd with the ultrasound scanner, his whoops of delight got more and more animated. All thirteen cows and heifers were pregnant and Chris could barely contain himself, exclaiming 'Chips and rice!' as the last animal ambled out of the crush and into the yard. I was not exactly sure why a double-carbohydrate meal should be a cry of celebration, but one thing was certain – there would be another successful generation on his farm the following summer.

Once suckler cows like these have been pregnancy tested, they don't usually need to see a vet.* They graze happily, patiently awaiting the arrival of their calves (a point at which a vet *might* need to be involved). But I had been to see Bertha a few times since the day of the pregnancy tests. She had a sore eye, which became a lingering problem over the course of several weeks. It was the lower lid that was causing the trouble. The surface was ulcerated, making the eye water and attracting nuisance flies, which increased the irritation and discharge still further. Chris had tried using various eye ointments, without success. The lack of improvement in his favourite cow was causing him increasing anxiety. The regularity of his messages to me, and the weekly photographic updates, signified his growing concern. It was a concern I shared.

I suspected it was a type of cancer called a squamous cell carcinoma. These are problematic cancers that can affect the white parts of cattle, particularly around the eyes. Given that *all* of Bertha was white and that this lesion had failed to heal with conventional methods, I feared the worst. The eyelids, and the surrounding skin, are particularly prone to squamous cell carcinoma. In cattle, it does not usually spread around the body, but does progress slowly, over months, gradually getting worse and

---

* Suckler cows, unlike dairy cows which see the farmer twice every day and sometimes the vet every few weeks, live an extensive life, grazing grassy pastures by summer and rearing their calves. They usually don't see much of the farmer and even less of a vet.

worse. Had it been on a different part of the body, or on a different species of animal altogether, treatment would have been simpler. Cats with white ears, for example, can get squamous cell carcinomas on the ear tips as a result of sun damage. It is the feline equivalent of skin cancer in people and can be prevented by applying Factor 50 sun cream. And for a cat that already has these tumours, the answer is to remove the ear tip. The cat looks odd without its pointy ears, but the surgery is simple and the cure complete. However, a squamous cell carcinoma in or around the eye, particularly the eye of a fully grown cow, represented a very much bigger challenge.

While I had got to know Bertha quite well, I knew Farmer Chris even better. I had been looking after his herd of cattle and his rare-breed pigs (Oxford Sandy and Blacks, otherwise known as Plum Pudding Pigs, on account of their brown colour and black spots) for about five or six years, ever since he had started his farm. His enthusiasm and passion for his animals was infectious and we immediately got on well. It is a joy for me to be around enthusiasts, no matter where the passion is directed, so I find it easy to connect with people like him. I had delivered Lucky, the last piglet in a litter, which had proved impossible for the farmer to deliver, stuck beyond Chris's reach. I'd vaccinated his stubborn horse, who hated vets and hated needles but liked jumping in the air and kicking forward and backward. I'd removed the huge horns from one of his splendid Highland cows. She was bullying the other (non-horned) cattle and needed tidying up to avoid a dangerous accident. I'd delivered calves in stressful situations in the middle of the night, and I'd trimmed the feet and removed the tusks of his cantankerous new boar, who was aptly named Donald, after the American president. The sedation I had to use to do this had temporarily – and completely accidentally – rendered Donald benign and mild-mannered, with absolutely no libido. I'd wondered if I should make a trip Stateside.

I'd also helped Chris inseminate his favourite sow, Elsie (although they all were his favourite), using artificial insemination. But that's a whole different story!

So, I knew my patient and her owner. I knew one of them was not getting better and I knew that the other one was very worried. Farmers are often perceived as tough, rough types, stoically out in all weathers and belligerently intent on keeping trespassers 'off my land'. The truth can be very different. Most are very attached to their animals. They worry about whether a treatment will be successful, and get upset if things don't go to plan. I was once called to see a cow that had fallen into the pit in the milking parlour. This is the area where the farmer stands to milk the cows. The pit is below ground level so the farmer's hands are at the same level as the cows' udders, making the job easier on the back. One of the cows, affected by milk fever, had wobbled, toppled and landed in this pit. It's a problem that I've only heard of happening once before, which is odd because you'd think it was a big risk for wobbly cows. I've seen drunk veterinary students falling into similar holes on many occasions, but only once a cow. After much treatment with calcium and several attempts to pull the poor girl out, it became clear that she had given up the ghost and there was no option other than to put her to sleep. As the final few millilitres of lethal injection ran into her jugular vein, the farmer, who had previously shown no trace of emotional connection with this or any of his cows, flung his arms round her neck and burst into tears, proclaiming his love and sorrow.

On another occasion, I went to perform a fertility test on a handsome new bull belonging to a farmer called Eric. The bull had been running with Eric's heifers, but when we came to pregnancy test them only a couple were in calf. This was a big problem, hence the need to check the bull's fertility. The procedure is simple enough, as long as you have the equipment and know what to do with it. A large, torpedo-shaped probe is inserted into the animal's rectum and gentle electrical pulses are applied to the prostate. Soon, an erection develops and moments later the semen appears, and can be caught in a test tube and analysed down a microscope. The process also allows examination of the bull's genitalia, which is important in case there are problems such as a bent or deviated penis. A bent or deviated penis will not cut the mustard.

In this case, the semen sample was perfect but the penis failed to emerge from the prepuce – a condition called, amusingly, short penis syndrome, which is an accurate description of the problem. While the semen was good, the bull was failing to put it where it needed to be, and this was the reason that hardly any of the heifers were pregnant. I explained this to Eric. The potentially prize-winning but, as it turned out, short-penised bull would need to be sent for T-bone steaks. He had no future in breeding.

At this time, I had just started my involvement with Channel 5's *The Yorkshire Vet* and the whole, sorry story of the bull with the short penis was filmed by an effervescent camera operator and producer-director called Izzie. She asked Eric about the implications of the bull's inadequacies and what it meant to him and the farm. To everyone's astonishment, Eric started to cry. Tears poured down his weather-beaten cheeks as he explained how upset he was; he was trying to improve his herd with this beautiful bull, but it was a case of one step forward and two steps back. Another tough farmer had been reduced to tears.

Chris was not quite at the point of tears over Bertha, but I sensed he was emotionally attached and I dared not contemplate what would happen if things did not go to plan.

I felt like part of Bertha's extended family, I thought as I examined her again, I had seen her so many times. The lesion on her eyelid had not responded at all to any of our previous treatment. I mulled over the options. I was looking at three possibilities:

A I could resect the whole of the lower lid. This would be relatively simple, but the healing would be awful and slow and painful. I felt the ongoing result would be inadequate and the eye pain would persist. Bertha would have to struggle without a lower eyelid, which would not be nice.

B I could euthanise Bertha. Sad as this option was, and not one that Chris would rush to take, it was a course of action that many commercial farmers would opt for. This simple solution would remove the pain and discomfort immediately.

C I could remove the eye in its entirety, along with the surrounding diseased tissue. This procedure would not be simple but, if successful, would offer a permanent solution. Bertha would be cured.

I reached a decision.

'Chris, we're gonna have to remove this eye,' I explained, as I reached out to scratch the unlucky cow on the forehead. My gesture of friendship didn't work – Bertha mistook my friendly hand on her forelock for another nuisance fly, intent on making her eye itch even more. She flung her head up and down and side to side, as if to disagree vigorously with my plan. I went through the options again with Chris, but knew that there was only really one way forward. Removing just the lower lid would leave a gaping hole and cause more problems than it would resolve and, happily, I knew there was no chance that Chris would opt to euthanise Bertha at this stage. The whole eye and all the surrounding tissues connected with the eye would have to be removed. I have done this procedure countless times on dogs and cats, and even rabbits and the occasional guinea pig. Commonly, it is carried out to resolve the chronic pain of glaucoma, where the build-up of pressure within the eye is unbearable; occasionally it is to deal with a cancer of the eye or its surrounding structures. The word used to describe removal of the eyeball is enucleation. When the eyeball and all its associated ocular structures – eyelids, tear ducts, lacrimal glands, muscles and fat connected to the eyeball and so on – are removed, the procedure is called extirpation, which is an excellent word and one you might expect to find describing some egregious punishment from medieval times. Usually, if a procedure has a complicated name, it means it is complicated to perform. This was no exception. It was going to be a complicated job and a fairly horrible one too. Removing any important part of the body is not something to which vets aspire. We like to save things, fix things, maintain a happy status quo. Removing Bertha's eyeball, and all the bits around it, would not be pleasant, especially since the eyeball itself was actually healthy.

It was a daunting prospect. To perform an extirpation on a cow is fraught with potential problems. Firstly, it is not possible to put a cow under full general anaesthetic, so I would have to sedate Bertha and infiltrate local anaesthetic to numb the area. She would need to stay completely still. I would need to perform quick and efficient surgery; I would need to avoid causing excessive bleeding; I'd need to excise every little last bit of cancer – even a small area left behind would render the whole procedure pointless. I would need to be as sterile as possible to prevent infection, and I'd need to keep her pain-free in the subsequent days. I was also anxious that, having resected the lower lid with a sufficient margin to remove all the bad tissue, there might not be enough skin to close the wound. I explained all this to Chris. He had turned a pale shade of green by this point, but nodded firmly.

'I feared that you'd say that,' he said, 'but the thing is, she's my favourite cow and I want to do everything I can for her.' Then he added, 'You couldn't just cut that bit off?', pointing at the sore lower lid.

It was my turn for firm head movements, but this time shaking rather than nodding.

'And there's no chance it might go away by itself?'

Again, more head-shaking from me.

'Tell you what,' I conceded. 'It's not urgent. Yes it's sore, but she's quite happy at the moment. Let's wait until she's had her calf. It will be one less thing to worry about and it saves putting her calf at risk.' I knew that this hard decision would become easier over the course of time, as it became clearer that the problem wasn't going to go away.

We didn't have to wait long. Just a week or so later my phone started to ping again with Chris's messages. Bertha had given birth to a lovely white calf, snowy white in fact, which was skipping around and full of health. We arranged a day and a time for the breath-holding operation.

Two weeks after the calf had been born, I returned to the farm. We had allowed sufficient time for the calf to take all the colostrum – the first milk, packed with nutrients and protective antibodies – that she needed. She was a strong calf and had a good start, so if the worst came to the worst and my surgery was a disaster, she would at least have a decent chance of surviving alone. But this was not my plan and I was reasonably confident it would go well. Chris was absolutely not confident and was visibly anxious when I arrived. He was, however, clear in his mind that something serious needed to be done. The tumour had got worse and it was obvious that it could not be put off any longer.

Bertha was already waiting in the pen and everything was ready. I explained my plan. We would get her in the cattle crush to keep her still and safely restrained. Then I would give her some sedative. It was important to get the dose right. Too little and she would fling her head around wildly, making the surgery impossible. Too much and she might collapse to the floor, again rendering it impossible to operate. Once she was sedated, I would inject large amounts of local anaesthetic around and behind her eyeball to numb the whole area. Next, I'd give painkillers and anti-inflammatories – they work better if they are administered in advance of the surgery. Then it would be time for the action proper. By the end of my explanation, Chris was looking ashen. It was hard to blame him. Over the course of the next forty-five minutes or so, I'd be removing the right eyeball from his favourite cow. It was likely there would be a lot of blood and there were, in truth, many things that could go wrong.

The sedation and administration of local anaesthetic went as I had hoped and, once I was happy Bertha couldn't feel anything, I took a deep breath and reached for my surgical instruments. The first part of the operation was to suture the eyelids together, smoothing out the skin above and below the eye. Next, I made a curved incision below the lower eyelid, where the tumour was. It was crucial to take a wide enough margin to ensure all of the cancer was removed. If any were left behind, then the whole procedure would be a waste of time. The second incision was above the eye, joining at either end onto the lower incision, making a scarlet ellipse. Next was the hardest part – dissecting out the whole eyeball; cutting and bluntly dividing the muscles that connect it to the inside of the bony orbit. These muscles are responsible for movement of the eye within its socket, and there are quite a lot of them. I was making steady progress, although blood seeped steadily from my op site and a large, red pool was congealing around my feet. Happily, Bertha was the perfect patient and had kept completely still during the procedure so far. My sedation and anaesthesia was spot-on. The increasing size of the pool of blood was not so spot-on, however, and I tried to conceal my concern. I reached for clamps and swabs and more clamps and more swabs, until I'd run out. I had to start recycling my clamps, ligating any vessels I could see as I went. Halfway through, my extirpation did, indeed, look like some kind of medieval massacre.

After what seemed like ages, the eyeball and its surrounding tissue finally came free and I dropped it on the makeshift operating table, which was made of a plank of wood on a wheelbarrow. I returned to the surgical site, which was still oozing. Suddenly, I remembered a spare packet of swabs I had in my car.

'Chris, can you go to my car and find a packet that looks like this?' I said, pointing to an empty autoclaved package sitting next to the eyeball.

He was clearly glad to have an excuse to vacate the grisly scene for a few moments, but there had not been much improvement by the time he reappeared clutching the packet of swabs. There was his favourite cow, missing an eyeball, with a huge bloody hole instead. Bertha would have won first prize in a Halloween competition. I told him how to open the packet without affecting its sterility and eventually, with the help of the extra swabs, the flow of blood abated. With huge relief, I started suturing up the gaping hole. With each suture, the situation improved. Bertha looked more like a normal cow and my stress hormones and blood pressure started to go back down. Chris regained the colour in his cheeks and started talking again. Finally, the last suture was placed.

Bertha's calf had been standing nearby in the adjacent field for most of the operation, as if she was supervising proceedings. Bertha would not have been able to see her, because her good eye (now her only eye) was looking into the cowshed, but once I'd unfastened her halter she swung her head round, caught sight of her calf and let out a massive 'moo'. It was time to let her loose and she staggered, still partly sedated, into the field to find her waiting calf. Chris and I watched as mum ambled and calf skipped across the paddock to a quiet corner. The calf nuzzled for a teat and we both looked on, relieved, from a distance as they reconnected. It was early days, but so far all looked good. We shook hands and crossed our fingers!

Chris sent updates every few days after the op, with photos and messages via my phone. Bertha was progressing well, but I could sense Chris was still worried. There was a lot of swelling. I reassured him that this was to be expected. I prescribed some more medication, hoping that time was all that was required. But after about three weeks, he asked me to call and see Bertha again, in person. I didn't know what to expect. Had the cancer returned? Was the wound okay? Maybe it had burst open, or perhaps she was suffering from all that blood loss? Maybe there was a huge abscess under my sutures.

I pulled into his farmyard with some trepidation.

'Thanks for coming, Julian. She's in that field,' Chris said, pointing to the paddock where all the other cows were grazing.

'How is she getting on?' I asked tentatively.

'Can you see which one she is?' he asked.

I surveyed the herd and had to admit I couldn't see her.

'That's the thing, Julian!' Chris exclaimed. 'You would not know she'd had anything done. That's her there.' He pointed at a cow with a spotlessly white calf suckling contentedly.

'It's totally amazing! Apart from having just one eye, you'd never know anything was wrong! It's totally amazing!'

I opened the gate and went into the paddock to get a closer look. The wound had healed perfectly and the hair was even growing back. Chris followed me, continuing to chat excitedly, using words like 'miracle' and 'amazing', before finally patting me on the back and saying, 'Thank you for saving my cow!'

I left him in the field, scratching his cow's back and admiring her calf, as the ubiquitous camera team set up their shot to interview him about how he felt about the operation and the outcome. As I leant on the gate, enjoying the last of the late summer sun, I could hear Chris uttering more superlatives. As the final few questions were asked, probing for an emotional reaction, I was sure I'd caught a glimpse of a tear in the corner of his eye. Another tough Yorkshire farmer had been reduced to tears of emotion. This time, at least they were tears of relief and happiness.

2. Dogs

There is something very special about the interaction between a human and a dog. It is a relationship, I would argue, closer and more powerful than any other. And it's a historic one, dating back fifteen thousand years, to a time when *Homo sapiens* was finding its feet and forming the ideas that would shape the future of our planet. In that pre-agriculture world, when our forefathers roamed the Earth hunting and gathering, and before we had domesticated any other creature, the dog appears to have joined our pack. Dogs assisted with hunting and fighting and acted (much as they sometimes do nowadays) as an early warning system if interlopers invaded the human groups. A tomb exists from around this time, in which a fifty-year-old woman was buried with her puppy, her arm resting on its little head. Dogs had integrated with humans, coexisting, communicating and co-evolving. Affectionate dogs, those attentive to the needs of primitive humans and the ones more adept at warding off predators probably received extra treats. Maybe dogs realised they were on to a good thing and developed the skills to manipulate their human hosts? A mutually beneficial relationship developed, and it was certainly one that would persist and become enhanced over the following millennia.

As a veterinary surgeon who works with dogs all the time, I see this relationship every day. It doesn't take a psychiatrist to spot the strength of feeling and the deep emotion that arises when a canine patient is sick. I don't usually give my clients hugs, but it can be a necessity at times when a beloved, lifelong companion is in a precarious place. I know farmers who think more about their collie than they do about their wife. The collie never moans or complains. There are women who are more connected to their Staffie than to their husband. The Staffie doesn't bugger off to the pub every night and his love is unconditional.

I experience the strength of the canine–human bond myself, with my faithful Jack Russell, Emmy. It was the same with our first dog, Paddy the cute-but-slightly-dim Border Terrier. Another Paddy (also a Jack Russell), along with his sister Sue and a Bedlington terrier called Judy, were my unswerving pals when I was just a toddler, so I've been immersed in dogs for all the time that I can remember.

The most complicated medical case I've every investigated and treated was in a Border Collie called Bobby. We were so close I felt we had become kindred spirits. I had to blood test him every few days to plot the cyclic changes of his blood cells in order to make a diagnosis of the rarest of conditions; I examined him on Sundays, even when I was not on duty, as my colleagues all knew I would rather treat him myself. I knew the vagaries of his condition and his personality so well. I'd given him countless injections to ease his headaches and control the overwhelming infections that threatened to swamp his depleted immune system. Despite me prodding him with needles every time I saw him, he would wag his tail, open his mouth wide as if smiling to greet me and lift his paw so I could take a blood sample or give him yet another intravenous injection. He was a patient and a friend.

I've spent my whole veterinary career treating creatures many and varied, and I'm often asked my favourite. It can be a close decision at times, but, when push comes to shove, give me a dog any day of the week.

The Hound of Gormire

M rs Davison walked serenely past me as I waited outside my consulting room for my next patient. She nodded her head politely in my direction. I had spotted her large dog, Bran, and her small husband a few moments earlier. Their progress had been anything but serene. Bran the Rottweiler, who was almost the same size as Mr Davison, had charged past me, briefly sniffing my crotch on the way, before bursting into the adjacent consulting room. In there, the worried senior vet of the practice was cowering behind his consulting table, hoping it would afford some protection. Mr Davison whizzed by, his mop of silver hair flashing like lightning in front of my eyes, travelling at the same speed as Bran but about two metres behind, clinging to the very end of his lead.

'Hello, Julian. Bran has come back for another check over. It's his heart, you know,' explained the elderly lady in hushed tones, as if not wanting the rest of the waiting room to hear the personal problems of her dog. I had not yet had the pleasure of meeting Bran in a professional capacity, and I was in no great rush to get up close with the ferocious Rottweiler. Fortunately, for now, this wasn't my concern. The elderly couple had been seeing my colleague for years and, despite the look of utter fear in the senior partner's eyes (which I could see from outside his room, some five metres away), he was stuck with the job of keeping Bran healthy. At least until such time as one of them (Bran or the vet) expired or retired. Judging by the alacrity with which Bran had just rushed past me and by the size of the new house that my boss had just purchased, there was no likelihood of either happening imminently, so he was stuck with a four-weekly heart check-up/encounter with danger for the foreseeable future. Of course, there was always the option of trying to persuade the Davisons to see a different vet, but this would not be easy either.

The door of the consulting room closed firmly, but it did little to muffle the sound of loud and testosterone-fuelled barking intermingled with nervous laughter. I smiled to myself and called in Barney the spaniel. I'd known this lovely dog since he was little and we were great friends. Safely in consulting room two, for once I felt I had drawn the long straw.

Barney was simple to examine and as friendly as usual – although his recently acquired habit of eating plastic flowers was proving irksome for his owner and also for me. I struggled to find any reason for this behaviour, but was considering either early onset senility or some sort of gastric irritation as the most probable causes. I dispensed a small, brown bottle of medicine to ease the soreness I had decided there must be in his stomach. I hoped the liquid would help, because there were no specific tablets to stop dogs eating plastic flowers. If this didn't work then I was at a loss. As Barney left, Bran was lurching out from next door. Froth and foam flew from the corners of his mouth like a rabid fox. There was no blood and I'd heard no screams, so I presumed his consultation had not ended in tears or death. Just as he had on the way in, and reminiscent of a scene from *Scooby-Doo*, Mr Davison followed at exactly the same speed, a lead's length behind. Mrs D chatted politely with the senior vet, who now looked more relaxed and was smiling and laughing. He'd escaped injury.

Mrs D smiled at me as she passed and said goodbye.

'That Bran is a bastard. I'm scared of him,' muttered my boss under his breath as he waved politely, smiling as the family went on their way. 'I'm not really frightened of many dogs, but that one has a nasty look in his eyes. I don't trust him.'

'How is he doing?' I asked. I knew Bran had a bad heart, but judging by the spring in his step he didn't seem to be too poorly. 'Have you done an ECG?' I was, and still am, very interested in cardiology and I took an active interest in every cardiac case that came into the clinic. However, in this case, it was a silly thing to say. I suspected I'd be throwing myself into a newly opened can of worms.

A few weeks later, I realised a plan had been hatched. It involved a house visit, an ECG machine and me. The plan wasn't a very subtle one.

'Julian, Mrs Davison has invited us both for tea at her house,' said my boss, lightly, as if he'd just remembered. 'She'd like you to get to know Bran. In case he ever needs treatment if I'm not around, on holiday or anything like that. Let's see if we can find a day next week when we're both available. And I'd like to do an ECG, to check his heart. Maybe you could help?'

This sounded like a pleasant idea, if one that really was rather strange.

The daily life of a busy vet usually precludes any opportunity to spend long, lingering afternoons drinking tea and eating cakes. To find the time and space in the diary for *two* busy vets to socialise in this manner would be almost impossible, but the boss was determined to find such a time. He even cleared my diary for me, something that had never happened before. He was very keen to get me introduced to Bran and his family over tea. Equally important was the fact that he had no idea how to attach the ECG leads to a patient or operate the machine, let alone interpret the patterns on the trace. As the self-appointed cardiac expert in the practice, I'd dropped myself right in it.

Two weeks later, the visit had been arranged and we readied ourselves for the afternoon tea appointment with possible death, me with the briefcase-sized ECG machine under my arm. Then, just as we were ready to leave, an emergency appeared. My boss, who would usually strenuously avoid an outside visit as darkness approached, suddenly became adamant that his surgical skills were essential to this case and rushed to attend an injured mare. He gave his apologies, scribbled directions to the Davisons' cottage on a scrap of paper, grabbed a stitch-up kit and headed out in the opposite direction. I felt I had been, or soon would, be like the injured horse: stitched up.

I followed the directions on my scrap of paper, heading up towards Sutton Bank then turning onto the winding lanes towards Gormire. It was already getting dark. In North Yorkshire in late November, the afternoons are short and the light doesn't last long. Making my way cautiously along narrow and deserted lanes, I could empathise with Watson and Holmes as they approached a different mire – Grimpen Mire – to solve the mystery of *The Hound of the Baskervilles.* Would I be able to solve the mystery of this hound's heart disease? The sense of foreboding grew as darkness fell. I didn't know exactly where I was going, but the scribbled map was good and eventually I arrived at the cottage where Mrs and Mrs Davison and, more importantly, Bran lived.

The cottage was small and unimposing, but the lights from

within looked warm and inviting. At least it wasn't made of gingerbread, so I felt slightly safer. However, that feeling of security was short-lived as I got out of the car to howling and furious noise from behind the leaded windows. I gripped my stethoscope more tightly. I didn't know if I was really expected to examine the hound this afternoon, meet him or just get to know Mr and Mrs Davison personally, but at least clutching my trusty stethoscope I had a kind of professional barrier. If the worst came to the worst, I imagined I could hold it out in front of my face, like a wooden cross before a vampire. And to attach ECG leads to his legs – would that even be feasible? It seemed an impossible task!

The noise coming from inside the house was a deep and terrifying bark from the depths of the dog, and I hadn't even yet knocked on the door. Bran was clearly on form as usual and it was hard to imagine that his heart was seriously compromised.

Mrs Davison came to the door, opening it with caution as she checked with her husband that the dog was restrained. Once it was established that Bran was, indeed, safely fastened in the kitchen, the door was opened wide. Mrs Davison was wearing a smart, long dress, her grey hair neatly in a bun that sat on the very top of her head.

'Oh, do come in Julian, it's so nice to see you. Thank you for coming,' she greeted me warmly and ushered me into the sitting room. 'Are you alone?' From under the kitchen door and between barks, I could see a tongue and strings of saliva. The tea was brought in by Mr Davison, this time stooped over a tray of tea and cake, rather than being pulled by a mad Rottweiler. I apologised for my colleague's absence, explaining that there had been an equine emergency. For now, at least, it was just Mr and Mrs Davison and me, with Bran safely out of the way. But for how long?

What followed was truly bizarre. First tea was poured, then cake offered, and then Mrs Davison delivered a lengthy soliloquy on each of the previous dogs they had owned. Occasionally Mr Davison would chip in, confirming just how special or idiosyncratic one or another had been. Next came a series of photos. I love hearing about people's animals and it is nice to look at photographs of pets, but one or two is usually sufficient. I smiled as politely as I could, and tried to feign interest in the endless list of unusual medical conditions that accompanied each past and deceased dog.

'Brian, get the portraits please,' instructed Mrs D, and I realised, with dread, that the family artwork was about to be unveiled. Brian Davison shuffled off again, returning with paintings – mostly in oil – by the armful, each of which was ceremonially displayed and explained. Every time Mr Davison left the room to bring more paintings or fetch more tea, Bran's ferocious barking would reignite, reminding me of the elephant who wasn't, thankfully, in the room just yet.

The afternoon wore on, with more tea and cakes, more stories and more paintings. When should I make reference to Bran, the ferocious hound in the kitchen, I wondered? Were they actually expecting me to perform an ECG? Did they even want me to examine him, or was this just a social occasion? It certainly seemed to be so far! More pictures of previous Rottweilers, all of which looked beautiful, calm and friendly. I wished any one of them was in the kitchen rather than Bran.

Eventually, I plucked up the courage to bring conversation round to the hound. If I had to examine him and assess his heart then I should get on with it. Risking my head being swallowed whole seemed preferable to yet another photo album.

'And how is Bran at the moment?' I ventured. 'I'd like to listen to his heart. And maybe perform an ECG. Would that be possible?'

'Well, Julian. That's a very good question and I'm so glad you've asked,' came the reply. Instinctively – more, induced by fear – I gripped my stethoscope. I felt myself beginning to cower on the chair, just like my boss had cowered behind his consulting table.

'Bran is doing very well indeed,' Mrs Davison confirmed. 'After he saw *his favourite vet*, last week, he's been absolutely fine. We won't need anything else until his next check-up in *four weeks' time*. Bran is looking forward to it already. You don't need to examine him this afternoon, Julian. But it would be *lovely* if you could say hello to him. Brian, bring him in to see Julian!'

I relaxed slightly, safe in the knowledge that I could get away with a less confrontational encounter with Bran. Moments later, Brian and Bran barged into the sitting room again. Saliva was spilling from the Rottweiler's gaping mouth, but at least he was on a lead. I tentatively held out a lowered hand, which Bran sniffed. He didn't try to attack me straight away, which I took as a bonus. Of course, he still made dangerous noises, but if I imagined very hard and squinted my eyes, I thought I could just about see the slightest hint of a wag in his stumpy tail. Much as the inquisitive cardiologist in me was desperate to attach leads to his legs and get a trace of his heart's electrical activity, my sense of self-preservation was stronger. I preferred to protect the electrical activity of my own heart.

We petted Bran (or as close to petting as is possible with a man-eater) for a few more minutes before Mr Davison went and sat with him metres away and finished his tea. Eventually, Bran was returned to the safety of the far side of the kitchen door. I sensed this was time to depart. Profuse thanks followed from both me ('thank you so much for inviting me for tea; thank you so much for letting me get to know Bran') and from Mrs Davison ('thank you so much for coming; thank you so much for taking the time to get to know our little Bran').

I headed for home, unscathed and relieved. I was mildly disappointed not to have checked the patient's heart but glad that I had not been dismembered by Bran, the Hound of Gormire Cottage. I was even more pleased that he would *certainly* be seeing my colleague next month and not me. It had been a great plan and a good try!

This Week I have been Mostly Sticking my Finger up Dogs' Bottoms

This week I have been mostly sticking my finger up dogs' bottoms. It sounds like a line from an episode of *The Fast Show* with Jesse the tramp – 'This week I have been mostly eating taramasalata', or 'This week I have been mostly eating roast chicken', or 'This week I have been mostly wearing nipple clamps' – all undoubtedly very funny. Hilarious. But sticking your finger up a dog's bottom is not at all funny, even if it sometimes feels as if it's what I do most. 'So why?', you ask. 'WHY?' There are a multitude of reasons why a vet needs to do this and the donning of a latex glove, followed by the liberal application of gloopy lubricant to the index finger and sometimes thumb, is something with which veterinary surgeons are well acquainted. It is not a very nice thing for the dog and it is not a nice thing for the vet, but it is important because it allows investigation of this part of the body. It can also offer a means of treatment in some cases, effecting a cure.

A rectal examination can detect all sorts of problems – prostate disease, hernias, growths and masses and, of course, the dreaded anal glands. These noxious structures are scent glands that sit either side of the anus, at approximately four o'clock and eight o'clock, if you imagine the anus as a clock face (don't dwell on that image though). These glands fill up with a horrible secretion, sometimes watery, sometimes pasty but always smelly, which usually empties when a dog passes faeces, and acts as a method of marking territory. Nowadays, dogs' territory is usually marked by the garden fence or the perimeter of the park around which they are taken for their morning walk, and the glands are largely redundant. They serve as a nuisance for everyone rather than offering any kind of benefit. They are a particular nuisance if they empty onto the sofa or car seat.

Sometimes the glands don't empty properly and the result can be impaction, which sounds like a condition from Herriot days. 'I think he has impaction of the anal glands, Mr Herriot' could easily appear alongside 'I think he has stagnation of the lung, Mr Herriot'. But it is a very common problem and probably one that has not changed at all over the years. The treatment is still the same in the twenty-first century as it was in James Herriot's post-war heyday.

A finger is inserted to allow palpation of each gland. They range from the size of *petit pois* in a small dog whose glands are relatively empty, to the size of a plump damson in a Great Dane whose glands are full. There is no need for complicated tests or MRI scans to diagnose this problem. Even before we insert the lubricated digit, the behaviour of the dog as described by its owner is usually enough to identify the problem.

'She's been scooting along the round and going mad with her back end,' is a common description. 'He can't stop licking under his tail,' is another. Either way, it is easy to diagnose impacted glands and also easy to fix. Squeezing each gland, with the index finger in the rectum and the thumb outside and (hopefully) catching all of the smelly contents in a wad of cotton wool, is one of the first things that veterinary surgeons learn to do. It is also one of the first jobs that senior vets learn to delegate to junior vets and that junior vets, in turn, delegate to students.

I can remember precisely my first brush with a dog's anal glands. I was an enthusiastic schoolboy, aged sixteen, eager to become a vet one day. Every Thursday after school I walked to the local veterinary surgery in Castleford and spent a few hours watching, learning and, where I could, helping out (there's not very much that a schoolchild can do to help, but it's important to get as much practical experience as possible before applying for a place at vet school). The evenings were long but full of interest and excitement and I would get home, well after eight o'clock, with aching feet from standing up, hungry for my tea and thirsty for knowledge. Most teenage boys fondly remember the exact details of their first kiss. In my case, it was my first anal gland encounter that I can recall in full, fetid detail.

I was just a bit *too* thirsty for knowledge as I leant in, peering under the dog's tail to get a better view. The vet, clearly without concern for the vet-to-be, gave not a hint of a warning as he squeezed the foul-smelling glands. A fountain of stinking, grainy liquid splattered my face, into my mouth and all over my hair. I tried to maintain my composure in this most horrible of circumstance, not wanting to draw attention to myself, as the grey goo congealed, infusing me with the unmistakable fishy aroma of dogs' bottoms. It stood me in good stead for the future. I treat the anal area of dogs with a healthy respect and I ALWAYS warn students to stand well back or to one side.

*   *   *

Those early pre-vet school days at the local practice were invaluable for me and really set me on the right track to becoming the vet I am now. I can still remember lots of the cases I saw, lots of experiences and, in particular, lots of the smells. The disinfectants, the surgical spirit and the peculiar smell of antibiotics were all new to me. At least they were better than the smell of anal gland contents. On one occasion a vet spent ten minutes during his busy surgery explaining to me all about a hormonal condition called 'Cushing's disease'. I diagnose this condition every month or so and its clinical signs are etched into my mind from that very first encounter.

One of my jobs on a Thursday evening was to count out tablets and put them into pots or packets. In those days, there was no proper system of checking or double-checking and it was all very relaxed. One cat with a cat bite, infected and smelly, needed some antibiotics. The elderly vet, with his long, white coat and with his spectacles perched on the end of his huge nose, dictated the dose and all the details for me to write onto the tiny label. This was a challenge in itself – there was a lot of information to fit into a small space and my writing was not neat. Nowadays the computer generates a label and everything is much more efficient (and readable), but in 1988 the clarity of the instructions was entirely dependent on a fine biro and legible handwriting. Once I had written on the label, I had to find the correct tablets and count them out, into the pot or envelope. It was easy enough, although what I didn't realise at this time was that Synulox tablets came in two strengths – two hundred and fifty milligrams (for dogs) and fifty milligrams (for cats). One poor cat returned the following week for a check-up.

'Well, he's not much better,' reported the exasperated owner. 'It's been a devil of a job getting these tablets into him. Even if I can fit one in his mouth, it's impossible for him to swallow it.'

I quickly realised my mistake and shrank into the corner of the consulting room. It was my second mistake in as many weeks. I would not be dispensing the wrong size tablet again, just as I wouldn't be standing in the firing line for another dousing in anal gland contents!

But back to the week in question, when I had been mostly putting my finger up dogs' bottoms. Anal glands were the main culprits. Some were full, some were not too bad, some were impacted, some had watery contents and some were empty and just needed to be checked ('Can you just check his glands?' is quite a common passing thought from an owner as the consultation draws to a close).

Unusually though, this week's anal issues also involved tumours. Three of the dogs in question had nasty growths up there. Lottie the Labrador was in for a second opinion and possible surgery to remove the offending mass. Anne, my wife – also a vet – was consulting too, and called Lottie in for her examination. She didn't like what she found and stuck her head out of the consulting room to find another vet to confirm what she thought. I was happy to oblige. The fat Labrador continued to wag her tail happily, despite repeated anal intrusion, but it was clear to both of us that this was a terribly large and almost certainly inoperable tumour. It was about the size of a tennis ball and extended inwards, upwards and outwards. We agreed that the next step should be a biopsy to identify the type of tumour we were dealing with, but it was hard to explain the severity of the situation to Lottie's owner, as there was not much to see from the outside. Instinctively, I felt I should offer him a glove so he could feel what we had felt (obviously, I didn't).

A Cavalier King Charles Spaniel was next. Fortunately his tumour was smaller and offered some hope of surgical success. I was getting good at this!

Another patient, later in the week, was an old friend. I had been looking after Daisy, the elderly spaniel, for many years. She had suffered for almost her whole life with terrible arthritis in her feet. It had taken months – if not years – of tinkering with her medication to get the painful condition under some sort of control. In the early days she would stand in the consulting room, shifting her weight from foot to foot, her eyes sad with the telltale expression of chronic and unrelenting pain. I had not seen her looking that unhappy for a few years though, and the regime we had settled upon was working a treat. At each of her regular check-ups, Colin, her owner, would always add, '. . . and can you check her A.Gs, Julian?'

'A.Gs' was Colin's abbreviation for anal glands, of course, spelt out in the same way as people use J.C. for Jesus Christ or O.J. for orange juice. I think he thought the abbreviation might mitigate some of the rudeness of Daisy's problem. On every previous occasion during Daisy's attendance at my clinic, evacuating her 'A.G.s' had been a simple enough job, but this time it was very different. Her right 'A.G.' was elongated, knobbly, firm and irregular, bearing all the hallmarks of yet another anal gland tumour – the third of the week! I relayed the worrying news of my rectal findings and we discussed her options. Colin was adamant, and I was in agreement, that to attempt surgery at her age and with her other multitude of problems would not be helpful. Daisy, just like Lottie, continued to wag her tail throughout. We decided upon a conservative approach. The thirteen-year-old dog did not need to be on the receiving end of my scalpel.

The next day, which was Saturday, I had two early morning conversations with friends about their dogs before I even got to work. As I was out on my morning dog walk, I ran into Linda.

Her elderly Border Terrier, Cookie, had no anal problems, but the seventeen-year-old had many other issues. The determined but mildly demented terrier stubbornly refused to follow the normal laws of Border Terriers, who tend to lose their marbles completely at around thirteen to fourteen. Cookie plodded on, somewhat confused but very happy. He reminded me of my gran.

Then, as I pulled out of my drive on the way to the surgery, Steve, one of my neighbours, flagged me down. I switched off the radio and wound down the car window. The conversation started off about the importance of catching up for a pint and our attendance at the Great Yorkshire Show the following week, before finally moving on to his dog Harry, who was a Labrador just as old as Cookie.

'Ey, what would you do about this dog o' mine?' Steve asked, scratching his head. 'He keeps peeing all the time, as he walks along. We had a flood in the kitchen this morning. He pees and he drinks and he waddles along, peeing. It's got worse in the last few days.'

I started asking a few questions about his drinking habits (the dog's, that is) to get a better idea of the problem, while glancing at the time. The waiting room would be filling up and I didn't want to be late.

'It's probably his prostate, Steve,' I explained, aware that Harry had not been castrated. Prostate enlargement could easily be the cause of all his problems. I glanced at my watch again. 'Tell you what, let's have a feel.'

I jumped out of the car, opened the boot, found my box of latex gloves and applied my trusty lubricant. Kneeling down on the grass of the village green, I set about yet another rectal examination, this one very impromptu and in the street outside my house. I was very glad I was a vet and not a doctor!

Nelly with the Elephant Legs

Anne and I had been treating Nelly for over a year. Anne was the first to tend to the veterinary needs of this feisty little Scottie dog. She had a growth on one of the toes of her front right foot. It had grown rapidly and had all the hallmarks of something sinister. Anne's instincts, honed over decades of treating dogs and cats, were that the toe should be amputated as soon as possible. The surgery went smoothly and Nelly's recovery was perfect. Analysis of the growth at the lab confirmed Anne's suspicions. It was a nasty tumour and its removal had been the best course of action. But there was a chance it might recur, so every month or so Nelly came in for a check-up, and that was how I got to know her and her owners, who were two sisters, very well. A year on and she had been doing superbly. The foot was great, the regional lymph node was normal and we dared to hope that she had made a full recovery. However, out of the blue, things took a turn for the worse. Nelly developed some vague, non-specific signs of illness – her eyes were gummy and she was reluctant to go for her usual walks. The stump of her amputated toe was fine, but something just wasn't quite right. Then, a strange thing started to happen. Her legs seemed to get fatter. It was subtle at first and only affecting the front legs, but as time went on all her limbs took on elephantine proportions. I measured them with a tape measure for confirmation of their increased circumference.

I was concerned this might be a condition called hypertrophic pulmonary osteopathy, otherwise known as Marie's disease. This is a bizarre syndrome whereby the bones of the front (and sometimes also the back) legs become painfully thickened, usually as a result of a mass of some description growing in the lungs. Nobody seems to know exactly why this happens and it is pretty rare, but is something always to consider in a dog like this. At vet school, rare conditions with complicated names and even more complicated pathology were usually hard to remember. But, for me, somehow this one stuck. I explained my concerns to Nelly's owners. Surprisingly, the peculiarity of the disease and its inexplicable pathogenesis didn't seem to cause them any extra concern. They just wanted their little dog to be better and were happy for us to do whatever was required. X-rays of Nelly's legs and also her chest would confirm or rule out the problem. I arranged to do these the following day. The waiting room had become a second home for both the Scottie and her devoted owners, so there was not a trace of worry on anyone's faces as the three waited to be seen.

The X-rays were conclusive and remarkable. Nelly did, indeed, have legs like an elephant. The cortices (the outside bits) of the bones in her front legs and feet were distended, irregular and bumpy, thickened in an unnatural way. The chest X-rays showed more bad news. There was an obvious, plum-sized mass sitting slap bang in the centre of the right lung lobe. Before I called her owners with the grave news, there was time to deliver a quick lesson to the less experienced vets in the practice. This was an excellent learning opportunity for my uber-enthusiastic younger colleagues, as the condition had a once-seen-never-forgotten appearance on the X-rays. I called anyone who was nearby to come and look at the dog and the images. First, to the assembled crowd, I showed the legs.

'What do you think of these radiographs?' I asked. There were various comments, some 'oohs' and some 'aarghs' and some scratching of heads. I pointed out the salient points – periosteal reaction on the bones of the antebrachium (lower limb) and also the metacarpals, with moderate soft-tissue swelling. There was more scratching of heads and some blank looks when I asked what the next test should be, and if anyone had any differential diagnoses (this is the phrase vets use to mean a list of possible causes). I felt like Dr Paddy, the radiology specialist at Cambridge Vet School who taught the student-me all I knew about interpreting radiographs. Unfortunately, Paddy's soft and lilting Irish accent, which drifted through the dimly lit radiography room like some ethereal spirit, also sent me into romantic daydreams. I could and should have learnt so much more from her brilliant teaching, if only I hadn't been thinking of other things.

'Julian, can you see the soft tissue density in the caudo-dorsal lung fields?' she'd ask, as sweetly as Tommy Shelby's wife, Grace, but my mind was elsewhere, in fields of a completely different kind. Luckily, as well as daydreaming about fields, I did also study hard in my radiology rotation and I've always had a passion for interpreting the black and white images. But, judging by the blank expressions on the young faces of my colleagues, they had not paid sufficient attention in their radiology seminars. They didn't have a beautiful Irish tutor, I suppose. I pulled up the chest X-ray with the obvious mass in the caudo-dorsal lung field. This was easy to spot, but still no one had made the connection between the dog, her legs, the first and the second X-rays. I made my pronouncement of the diagnosis. There was a quiet murmur of recollection from the depths of someone's veterinary memory, but I was, apparently, revealing to others a previously unknown disease. I pointed everyone in the direction of the textbooks.

Some years later, one of my colleagues, Candela, who was at this session, always sends me a text message whenever she encounters references to Marie's disease. So far, I've refrained from messaging Paddy whenever I make the diagnosis. But now I needed to report the news to Nelly's owners.

'What can we do?' was the obvious question. I went through the limited options and recommended a course of steroids in the short term. I hoped this would shrink both the legs and the mass. Nelly was already old and this was the second major problem she had developed. But the big question remained: could I remove the tumour?

Usually, a plum-sized mass is a simple thing to resect. But, when that mass is inside the chest cavity, in the middle of the lung, the procedure is a whole different ball game. Moreover, cancer in the chest is often a secondary and the result of metastatic spread. There may be other tumours, maybe invisibly small, in the lungs or other places like the brain.

The steroids helped for a week or so, but their potent effects quickly subsided. At this point, surgery to remove the lung lobe containing the tumour was the only course of action left. It was serious surgery, not for the faint-hearted and without any guarantee of success. After some further discussion, we all agreed it was worth the considerable risk. If the surgery went well Nelly could be cured. Without it, she couldn't continue. When put in such bleak terms, the decision seemed simple and we arranged a time for the operation.

A thoracotomy and lung lobectomy was pencilled in for the following week and big stars were placed all over the daybook to alert nurses and reception staff not to arrange any other procedures for the same day.

Not many lung tumours are amenable to surgery. Most of them spread rampantly through the lung tissue, with secondaries seeded everywhere. They are usually associated with serious breathing problems and the prognosis following intervention can be terrible. But Nelly was different – her lung tumour was not actually affecting her respiratory system at all. Just her painful, elephantine legs and her disposition.

There was a palpable tension in the air on the day of surgery. Nelly was oblivious but her owners were worried. So were all the staff. It was all hands on deck. Anne was there to help with the surgery, while two nurses dealt with the anaesthetic. Because the lungs would collapse as soon as we went into the chest cavity, Nelly would need to be ventilated manually throughout. One nurse would maintain the anaesthetic while the other took care of breathing for the little Scottie. I opened the ribs, using special retractors and sutures to get greater access to the lungs. The tumour was sitting there, just as it appeared on the X-ray, circumscribed and red, right in the middle of the lung lobe. Beside it, although moving rather than sitting, was Nelly's heart, beating and wobbling rapidly. It was a disconcerting sight. Under normal circumstances this is a part of the body that vets can only hear, using a stethoscope, or see with the help of an ultrasound or X-ray. To see it beating, the very essence of life itself, millimetres from my fingers – and worse, my scalpel and needle – was somehow exhilarating. Proper, human cardiac surgeons do things that are altogether more spectacular than what I was hoping to do today, but I – a mixed practitioner – would be at my technical limit. My plan was to remove the whole lobe, with the tumour in its centre.

At various points there were gasps, sharp intakes of breath and the occasional swear word from everyone in theatre. I had to bark instructions at Fiona, the nurse who was ventilating Nelly, as to when to give her a breath and when not to, so the inflated lung tissue didn't push her heart towards my sharp needle. I apologised afterwards for being bossy. Finally, the lung with the pesky tumour in its centre was out of the dog and on my surgical drape. There was still work to be done, as we sealed the chest wall and reinflated Nelly's lungs. Then it was the moment of truth, as Fiona stopped ventilating and we waited for Nelly to take her first breath unaided. It wasn't just Nelly who needed to breathe. As her ribcage rose and dropped by itself, there was a communal sigh of relief. It was done and, despite everyone requiring extra blood pressure medication, everything had gone very smoothly. As I placed the final sutures in the skin I said, 'it's just like that song by CamelPhat.'

Of course, I meant their recent hit single called 'Breath' rather than the previous one, which was called 'Panic Room'.

Nelly went home the next day, to the delight of her owners. She wagged her tail and, other than the huge bald patch on her right side, you would have never known that she had had part of her lung removed. Anne and I saw her again the following week for a check-up, by which time her legs had shrunk completely back to normal. She had responded better than anyone could have hoped. As her owners and I both agreed, she was a true 'miracle dog'.

Reel Around the Fountain

Lunchtime was, as usual, a brief affair, and I only just made it back to the practice in time to start my afternoon list of consults. I hurriedly shoved the remains of my panini into my mouth as I peered at the computer screen to see what the afternoon had in store for me. The first two appointments on the list looked as if they would be relatively simple, but the third looked anything but straightforward. In fact, it sounded positively clandestine, until I remembered an earlier conversation with Fiona, our vet nurse who had arranged the irregular consultation.

At half past two Jack, the 'Something-a-poo', was booked in for his regular and life-preserving injection. Jack had a serious illness that necessitated an injection once a month. He also had a needle phobia. This was a big problem and, in an attempt to solve it, Jack's owners had sought the advice of a pet behaviourist. The solution, according to the behaviourist, was to meet at a venue remote from the veterinary surgery, thus avoiding the negative association between the surgery and the injection. A plan had been hatched, therefore, for me to meet Jack in a car park somewhere between Boroughbridge and a small village called Scotton, in the middle of Nidderdale. In theory, at least, this was a sound plan. In practice, I had no intention of meeting a lady and her fluffy dog in a random and remote car park. People might talk.

So, the venue of the liaison was changed. The new plan was that I should meet Jack and his owner in the middle of Boroughbridge, next to the fountain. The appointment list on the computer gave the owner and the dog's details and, in the next column, where it would usually say *'booster'* or *'express anal glands'*, it said: *'meet at Fountain for injection'*.

It isn't actually a fountain because no water comes out of it. It looks more like a very small and therefore useless bandstand. Nevertheless, it made a convenient rendezvous point. I spotted Jack, waiting beside a bench with his owner, who was armed with a large block of cheese – apparently the weapon of choice as advised by canine behavioural therapists. The idea was that the tasty cheese would distract the dog from his fear of needles. Small morsels of sausage also, apparently, work. For my part, I was armed with a small syringe filled with Jack's powerful medicine, which I had surreptitiously hidden in my coat pocket.

We met and chatted, we ruffled ears and we shared a few crumbs of Cheddar on the bench, calmly getting to know each other before getting down to business. I'd met Jack just twice before. The first time was when we were in the process of making his diagnosis. He had a condition called Addison's disease, presumably first identified by a Doctor Addison (its more scientific name is hypoadrenocorticism). This is a complicated disease. It manifests itself in a multitude of ways and it's notoriously hard to diagnose. The signs are caused by a deficiency in the functioning of the adrenal glands. These crucial glands, each of which sits neatly behind each kidney, make various vital hormones:

adrenalin – the 'fight, flight or fright' hormone that comes into play when we are attacked by a pack of lions and allows us to run like the wind; cortisol – the hormone that allows us to cope with stress; and a third stress hormone called aldosterone, which has various effects on the kidneys and circulatory system. A failure of function in the outer bit of the adrenal gland results in production of insufficient cortisol and aldosterone and the consequences can be catastrophic. Collapse, kidney failure, reduced cardiac output, vomiting, abdominal pain and death are all signs. Milder cases present as vague illness, classically waxing and waning and lacking clear indicators. One common feature, however, evident in both mild and severe cases, is a slow heart rate, caused by elevated potassium levels.

Any vet student, or even budding vet-student-to-be, who is reading this chapter should log this disease in the back of their mind, ready to recall it if ever they see a poorly dog with vague signs and a slow heart rate. Although, any vet student will know that these are also classic signs of hypothyroidism. One should never jump to diagnostic conclusions without a proper set of tests, but without some form of pattern-recognition process, the path to achieving a diagnosis is tortuous. (The issue of pattern recognition in aiding a diagnosis is a different topic altogether.)

The second time I'd seen Jack was to start the series of regular injections, which would replace the hormones in which he was deficient, and without which he would not be able to survive. I hadn't seen him since then, as colleagues had taken over control of the maintenance of his condition.

In the 'olden days' (in my third decade of practising as a vet, I think I am just about entitled to use this phrase) there was a superb tablet for treating Addison's disease. It came in stumpy brown glass bottles, each with an unassuming khaki and white label. Each bottle held, inexplicably, just thirty little, life-saving tablets. Given that most dogs would need between five and ten tablets per day, each bottle lasted less than a week, which was not very environmentally friendly. The recycling bin filled very quickly. Despite its diminutive packaging and its benign name, which was full of soft sounding letters like 'f's, this drug kept many dogs with this unusual condition alive and healthy. Sadly, it was discontinued a few years ago and a new drug was produced, with a sexy name full of 'z's. Modern drugs nearly all have sexy names including lots of 'z's, 'x's and 'v's. This particular one comes only as an injection, which is even more sexy if you're a pharmaceutical company; injections can be sold to vets at a higher price than tablets and vets, in turn, charge more for injections than they do for tablets (which, these days, can be purchased almost anywhere, with or without authorisation or prescription). Injections, however, are not so sexy if you are a needle-phobic dog like Jack.

What Jack's behaviourist had failed to take into account was that a needle is a needle, whether it is in the surgery, in a car park or by the fountain. Even though Jack was calm and free from the stress of the veterinary clinic, he quickly realised what I was up to, spat out his cheese and spun round, intent on avoiding my syringe. I have administered hundreds of thousands of injections to animals over my career and, I have to say, I'm pretty good at it. I reckon it's one of my stronger points as a vet. Yes, I'm also a dab hand at spaying a bitch, emptying anal glands and lambing a ewe, but my injection technique – nay, style – is right up there. So, I managed to inject the medicine safely and effectively. But poor Jack spent the next few minutes rolling on the ground in anguish and distress, not even slightly mollified by the cheese that was supposed to distract him. The plan had clearly not worked at all and I did not fancy any more al fresco meetings like this. For the vet, dealing with a wriggly dog is much easier in the consulting room than it is in an open space and, for Jack, the experience had not been any better than it would have been in the clinic. His owner was palpably disappointed. I racked my brains for another solution. Then it struck me. The solution was staring me in the face and, ironically, it wasn't a solution at all. It was a tablet.

'You know, there might be another way,' I ventured, explaining my flash of inspiration. 'There is a tablet that we used to use for treating this condition. It's not available any more in this country, but let me see if I can find any online. If so, I'll get as much as possible. Then Jack won't need any more injections.' I didn't know whether I would be able to find any but it was worth a try. 'We used to use them in the olden days,' I added, trying not to sound like a vet from prehistory. I just hoped there were some of the magical tablets somewhere out there and available to purchase. It would save Jack's monthly trauma and save me any more clandestine meetings by fountains or in car parks. In a modern world, with sexy injections with fancy names full of 'z's, it's worth remembering that sometimes the old treatments, in small, brown bottles, are still the best.

'I Think it's a Bloody Version of . . .'

Dave the sheep farmer was larger than life and old-fashioned but wise, in his own way, and never without a weird or wonderful theory. He tended to a flock of a few hundred sheep and some miscellaneous cattle. He also had a couple of Border Collies that helped out on the farm, rounding up sheep and sometimes, but not always, assisting with the handling of Dave's cattle. On more than one occasion, however, I'd seen the dogs prove to be very much less than helpful. This was like most of the stuff on Dave's farm, which was supposed to make farming life easier, but often didn't. His cattle crush was rusting into the ground where it stood, grass emerging through the friable, rotten wood that had once been a floor. His cattle wagon, once used for transporting cattle to the fat stock sales at Thirsk market, or from the store sales at the markets in Northallerton or Skipton, sat inert with flat tyres and a peeling exterior, neglected and redundant. The buildings, once (about a hundred and fifty years ago) state-of-the-art, now were dark, dingy and dilapidated. Functional, but only just.

The low roof of the fold yard made it very difficult to clean out using a tractor, so Dave added clean straw on top of what was already there. This is a perfectly acceptable method up to a point (it is called a 'deep litter system' and usually provides warm, clean and comfortable housing), but on this farm the bedding got deeper and deeper as the winter progressed. The result was a straw bed so deep that it was impossible to enter the buildings without stooping. There was definitely less head space for the farmer when he checked his cattle as the winter season progressed. And by mid-March, even the cattle needed to stoop. When I visited to treat a heifer with pneumonia or a sheep with a prolapse, it was a constant challenge not to bang my head on the wooden beams and low brick archways. Add to this the tenacious nature of the manure underfoot and I considered it a victory if I could get to the patient, let alone make it better.

On one occasion, we had been struggling for some time in the gloom, trying to catch a sheep with a vaginal prolapse. The stooped and swearing figure of Dave, huffing and puffing, finally managed to capture the heavily pregnant ewe by her horns. Just as he turned her round so the grapefruit-sized, pink vaginal prolapse was pointing towards me, his trousers – which I can only assume had been held up with worn-out baler twine – fell down. Right to the floor. It wasn't a pleasant sight. Dave was not keen to let go of the sheep that had been so hard to catch, so he left his trousers where they were – around his ankles. An unhealthy image was burned onto my retinae, remaining there for the duration of my treatment of the ewe. It should not be described here.

But his dogs, although relatively useless at rounding things up, were well loved. Loved in a rugged, tough, sheep-farmer-whose-trousers-fall-down kind of way. I could not imagine many evenings when Dave would snuggle up with his collies on the sofa, rubbing them behind the ears or tickling their tummies, but nevertheless it was a love of sorts. So when I saw Dave leaning against the reception desk at the surgery, just before closing time on a Saturday morning, with one of his collies on a string, I knew it must be serious. The coffee for which I had been longing since I'd started consulting some hours previously would have to wait.

'Ah! I'm glad it's you,' called Dave, as he ambled down the waiting room with his dog, its tail wagging as it walked along, faithfully following on a bit of string. 'This 'ere dog o' mine has got summat up wi' its leg.' It was hard to say who was more lame – the dog or the owner.

Before I could invite him into the consulting room to find out the name of the dog (in fact I don't think it had a name – at no point did Dave call it anything other than 'this 'ere dog' and the clinical notes, in the end, simply said 'Farm Dog'), and before I could ask any further questions, Dave launched into a detailed description of what he thought about the cause of the lameness and the reason for the swelling, which was at the top, near his shoulder.

'This dog is lame,' he declared. 'He's not painful. Not at all painful, in fact. He still works the sheep like a good 'un, so he can't be in any sort of pain. I think . . .' (I sensed one of Dave's tangential theories was about to come out of his mouth), 'I think it is an abscess.' He paused, either expecting immediate agreement from me, the vet, or to take a breath before continuing to justify his theory. It turned that it was the latter, as he went on to explain his treatment of the supposed abscess: 'And so I've been injecting him wi' some penicillin. Every week. It's getting better, but it's still not right. What do you think?'

Before I could answer his question, which I considered was surely not rhetorical, he continued, ''Cos I think it's a bloody great abscess. In fact, I'm certain it is. It's just like a bullock I had a few years ago. Its leg was bloody swollen and I kept injecting it and, do you know what, it bloody went and got better. All the vets at this practice said I was wasting me time and that it was a job for the knacker man, but it came right. In the end. It came right in the end, it did. I think this lump is the same.'

I didn't feel like opening the can of worms that was the case of the lame bullock, and it was hard to comment on a historic case without proper knowledge. However, I could not agree with Dave's diagnosis in the case of the lame collie. I was as certain that this *wasn't* an abscess as he was certain it was. The firmness and size of the swelling, along with its position at the top of the left humerus, just below the shoulder, suggested it was actually a tumour in the bone, probably one called an osteosarcoma. The prognosis was grave and it was not something that would be improved by a few injections of penicillin. It wouldn't be cured by *any* injections, and my skills of tact and diplomacy were more important than my clinical skills if I were to persuade Dave that we weren't dealing with an abscess.

I examined the leg and discussed the possibilities, before recommending that we should take some X-rays under sedation to ascertain the nature of the swelling. Bone tumours have a very distinctive radiographical appearance and the sooner they are identified the better. Although the prognosis is poor, there are some treatment options available. I knew that the management of this leg would be palliative until the dog's quality of life deteriorated, but I still needed those X-rays to take away the guesswork and give us an actual diagnosis rather than Dave's conjecture.

But Dave was having none of it! He didn't know anything about X-rays or bone tumours but he knew everything about abscesses. He point-blank refused to let me do the tests.

Frustrated, I dispensed a pot of strong painkillers, hoping this would help. I asked the pair to come back a week later so I could do a follow-up.

However, a few weeks passed before Dave reappeared. It was another Saturday morning, around the same time, but this time he didn't bring his faithful hound. He wanted some Vetrap – a stretchy kind of bandage, usually used for bandaging the limbs of dogs or horses. From my position in the office, I could just make out the one-sided bargaining going on as Dave tried to get some money knocked off the price, based on a bulk buy.

'What do you need all this for, Mr North?' asked our diligent receptionist, Sylvia.

'It's to stop me bloody ribs from falling apart,' explained Dave. So he was intending to use the veterinary bandages to treat himself. I thought I should intervene at this point. I decided not to probe to deeply into the farmer's plan of self-curing. He thought he knew best and I had to pick my battles carefully. I wanted to find out about the poor dog. The tumour was likely to be painful, and I wanted to encourage the stubborn farmer into the correct course of action.

'How's the dog, Dave?' I asked, keen to start a dialogue that would persuade Dave to bring the canine patient, who still had no name, back to see me.

'Yer know what? It's *a bit* better. Not a lot, mind. I give him those tablets – I'm not sure they do a lot o' good, to tell yer truth. But I do inject him with that creamy antibiotic I have for the bullock. I still have a bit left and I *think* it's working.' My heart sank.

'And I'll tell yer summat else. I'm not sure this thing is an abscess after all. And do you know what I think this is?'

I dreaded what was coming next.

'I think this is a version of . . .'

I waited, hanging on Dave's enthralling words, for his amazing diagnosis.

'I think this is a bloody version of *wooden tongue*,' he proclaimed, pausing as if awaiting for a celebration from me that we finally had the answer.

But, since 'wooden tongue' is a chronic infection that affects the tongues of cattle, it was definitely not the cause of the collie's swollen leg. I was never going to be able to agree with the farmer's rustic and incorrect conclusion. Cows with the disease develop a progressive hardening of the tongue, as a result of a chronic infection by a bacterium called *Actinobacillus lignieresii*, which invades the tongue via minor abrasions from chewing wooden things or tough barley awns. Fibrosis develops as well as infection and the result is a tongue that resembles, well, wood. Affected cattle struggle to both eat and chew the cud so weight loss ensues, which can be fatal. It's uncommon nowadays, but back in the first years of my career, when cattle were surrounded by wooden feed troughs and wooden fencing, it was a condition we would see every few months. Treatment with drugs such as Dave's creamy antibiotic or huge syringes full of sodium iodide were often effective, but it wasn't a quick cure and cases often took months to recover. I hoped Dave was not planning to embark on any such treatment and I urged him to bring the collie to see me. However, much as he loved his dog, he did not like detailed diagnostic tests, so persuading the farmer to allow me to do a full work-up to confirm the tumour would be hard. Then I had an idea.

'Can you bring him in, Dave?' I suggested, 'I've never seen wooden tongue in a dog. It would be very rare. I'd like to take some X-rays, you know, just to check?'

'I'm not so sure about X-rays, they sound expensive. But I have 'im in the Land Rover if you want to have another look at 'im,' he muttered. While I was very worried about the collie and its future, Dave was clearly not and it had not even occurred to him that there was any need to bring him into the practice today.

'Yes please. I'd like to see him again. And there's no charge for the examination, so don't worry about that,' I offered, desperate for another chance to persuade the stubborn farmer into a diagnosis and the correct form of treatment.

But, it was the same all over again. The collie hopped in to see me, wagging his tail vigorously. The upper leg was very similar, with a huge, firm swelling, and I tried again to convince Dave to let me take an X-ray. Again, my persuasion failed. I reached for another tranche of painkillers and arranged for another check-up in a week.

It raised an interesting point about tests and consent. I was pretty certain that the mass was a tumour, but would an X-ray confirm that? It probably would, but standard practice would also require a biopsy to allow histological analysis (looking at the cells and the tissue structure down a microscope). This would take two full weeks, as the lab would need to dissolve the calcium structure of the bone before it could examine the cells. Even if I did all the tests, it was clear that whether it was a tumour, an abscess or even a bloody version of wooden tongue, Dave would not opt for invasive surgery and therefore management would be palliative to relieve pain and improve comfort. If the dog-with-no-name was happy, wagging his tail, eating his food and wanting to round up sheep, should we euthanise him simply because of the result of the X-rays, the blood tests or a biopsy? It is a tricky issue, made trickier with a stubborn farmer and no proper diagnosis.

I spent a month in a veterinary hospital in America when I was a student. I can still hear the words of the superb clinician, from whom I learnt a great deal; 'treat the patient, not the test results'.

Of course, he didn't mean we should ignore the test results, but that clinicians should make our judgements with the patient and its condition at the forefront of our minds. It was an important lesson. An inoperable chest tumour is bad, but don't reach for that final injection if the cat is happy. Euthanasia is first and foremost to relieve suffering, and it is crucial to make that final decision at the correct point. Clearly, Dave's dog had a big problem, regardless of what my X-rays might tell me, but it was also evident that he was still enjoying life and clearly Dave was not ready, and did not think it was the right time for euthanasia. So, in fact, X-rays or not, Dave would be taking his collie home until that point arrived.

That point arrived sooner than Dave had expected, because he was back before his next scheduled appointment. He drew up in his vehicle at the side door of the practice and carried his dog in.

'This 'ere dog. It needs putting to sleep,' he said in a rush, so as not to dwell on the emotion. 'He's not so good. He didn't 'ave his breakfast and his tail stopped goin' today, so I'd like you to put him down.'

I got some help from a nurse and gathered my equipment. As I returned to the consult room, I was sure I noticed Dave wipe away a tear from his eye. It is always a sad time, but outward displays of emotion from otherwise rough, tough adults make everything worse. It went smoothly and the collie who I thought had no name went straight to sleep.

'Thank yer for doing that, Julian,' Dave said as he scooped his dog up from the table and headed for the door to take him home to bury on the farm. 'It is sad but it was the right thing to do.' I nodded in agreement, for once.

Dave sniffed away more emotional tears as I held open the car door.

'Come on Tip, let's take you home. You've been a grand dog.'

I realised Dave, the stubborn old intransigent farmer, had more feelings for his dog than I had imagined. It was also then when I realised that the collie had had a name after all.

'And do you know what?' Dave added, still manfully sniffing back his tears as he climbed into his Land Rover with Tip for the final time. 'I think this bloody leg was some sort of bloody tumour.'

3. Pigs

The first photographic evidence that suggested I might devote my life to animals was a picture of me as a toddler, standing in front of my proud grandfather, clutching a piglet in my arms. Of course, when I was two years old, nobody knew that I would become a veterinary surgeon when I grew older and wiser, let alone find myself writing the introduction to a chapter about the very same animal with which I was first photographed. And, as coincidence would have it, on the very day of writing this introduction, I have spent a happy half-hour talking about and watching five litters of piglets with their mothers, on a sunny and still spring day.

Nowadays, as you will discover later in this section, vets in mixed practice hardly ever see individual pigs. Treating pigs is a specialist job, and is mostly done on a whole-herd basis. Even most pig specialists don't see many actual pigs, so I was very lucky. The practice where I was working had recently acquired a tranche of new farm clients because a neighbouring practice had given up its farm animal work. I was called by one of these new clients to see a lame sow, and I jumped at the chance to travel to the picturesque (but much derided by Harrogate panto-mime dames) village of Spofforth. Gary the farmer was waiting for me in the dusty lane and led the way to the pig pens. It was far from a commercial pig farm. Gary just kept a few pigs along-side the rest of his enterprise. It used to be a common thing for there to be a sow, whose snout would appear over a shed door as you drove into the farmyard. The practice died out for a while but, happily, a few more farmers have started to embrace the idea of keeping a couple of pigs again over recent years. I leant on the wooden door to the open sty and waited for my lame patient to appear from the arc at the far end. She didn't emerge, so Gary went to get food.

'There's not much a pig doesn't do for food,' he explained and soon, as predicted, the sow hobbled out of her arc, closely followed by another sow from the neighbouring pen who, sensing an extra meal might be on the cards, left her suckling piglets and jumped up at the gate, so her head was at exactly the same height as mine. Her open mouth, interested ears and small but glinting eyes told me everything about her inquisitive and cheeky personality. It was as if she was jumping up to say 'hello'. A scoopful of pig nuts kept her quiet while I examined her lame friend.

It turned out to be quite straightforward to treat, which gave me the opportunity to chat to the farmer, who was genuinely passionate about his livestock, to acquaint myself with his farm and, more importantly, watch his three-week-old piglets play in the sun. I'd forgotten just how amazing these stocky little bullet-shaped creatures are. Three were playing hide-and-seek, using their mother as cover. Two peeked out at me, cheekily, from behind a board and squealed with excitement when I looked directly at them. Another skipped over to the water trough where his mum had just been. He sniffed at and drank some water, then stuck his stumpy snout into the mud, sneezed and scuttled back to his siblings. Yet another little piggy clung tenaciously to one of Mum's many teats, trying to grab a snack as she wandered around her pen, looking for the warmest corner to lie down. Each piglet, identical in appearance, shape, size and colour, had its own fascinating and curious personality, if only we had sufficient time to observe and compare them.

But somewhere along the line, from a time when everyone had a pig in their backyard to modern-day commercial pig production, pound signs started to appear more prominently than they did in other areas of farming. They were almost slap-marked onto their bristly pink sides. In the first few paragraphs of *The Pig Farmer's Veterinary Book*, the words *cost*, *value for money* and *efficiency* are omnipresent. The very first sentence of the text in the inset of the cover states: 'This is a book that should pay dividends in the hands of any pig farmer. In the course of a few years it should recover its cost many times over, even in the most fortunate and best-managed herds'. The book was a present from my mother to her father (my grandfather, from the photo of us and the pigs), and it cost sixteen shillings. The inscription inside said: '*Love from Catherine, December 1961*'. It highlights the financial pressures of pig farming as far back as sixty years ago. Amidst this financial pressure, the poor, individual pig, its health and welfare stood little chance of retaining an identity. Perhaps it is because piglets are so similar to each other, so numerous and so good at growing, that their strengths as individuals, their personal traits and characteristics have been overlooked by the juggernaut that is the pig-farming industry. They have become an amorphous mass of pink, fleshy porcine growth statistics.

'We are all individuals!' they should shout, to borrow a line from Monty Python's *The Life of Brian*. Today though, in the spring sunshine of Spofforth, the piglets didn't need to shout anything. In the half-hour that I enjoyed watching them play their games, it was abundantly clear that pigs were all individuals. This next section is dedicated to the *individual pig*. Long may they continue, because the world seems a better place with a pig.

All Sorts of Farmers

I have met a lot of farmers over the years. While they certainly have many traits in common, they are a varied and disparate group and never fail to surprise me. At one end of the spectrum there are the round, red-faced, Range-Rover-driving types, often with an ego and a bank balance as big as their paunch. Hard work and an ability to spot an opportunity – in potatoes, poultry or fattening cattle – have paved the way for a comfortable lifestyle and a personalised number plate to adorn their shiny 4x4. My favourite of these number plates was one I spotted outside an auction venue, where I was occasionally called to attend to an injured animal that had slipped while rushing down the race, or as it came off a wagon. The number plate, which presumably belonged to a wealthy sheep dealer, was 'ewe 2'. I imagined someone in dark glasses with a band in tow. But farmers usually work alone and rarely wear dark glasses. In fact, close inspection of the vehicles at any busy livestock market in my part of the world reveals that quite a lot of farmers have private number plates. Far from this being seen as a frivolous and unnecessary expense – and I could write a whole book on how Yorkshire farmers are averse to unnecessary expense – a fancy number plate seems almost to be compulsory. I noticed one recently on an elderly and battered Land Rover Defender. Defenders were once a trusty workhorse, but are now often a customised fashion accessory for any countryman with more money than sense. This one, though, was not fancy and pulled a dilapidated sheep trailer. The number plate was 'X5 RAM', giving the impression that this farmer's male sheep were five times more potent, virile and meaty than any others. Looking round the car park at Thirsk Auction Mart, it seemed that number plates ending with 'COW' must be the cheapest, as these were most common on rusting Toyotas or Mitsubishis. The smartest vehicles, in the reserved spaces nearest the entrance, had the farmers' initials as plates. The F-type Jaguar, parked closest to the front doors, had not a speck of cow muck on it, but everyone inside the building knew who owned it: the man who had brought three lorryloads of fat cattle to sell that day.

At the other end of this farming spectrum is the pig farm worker. I can say this without being derogatory, because my grandfather, who was a great and honest, hard-working and loving man, kept pigs. With his flat cap, engrained with both the odour of pigs and the fine, dusty particles of milled pig food, and his overalls with straps buckled over his broad shoulders, he looked (and smelt) like a typical pig man. Being a pig man is a hard life, but you rarely hear a word of complaint, because, almost without exception, pig men love their pigs.

Ivan Stubbs was a pig man struggling to make a basic living. He had a herd of commercial sows and their fattening offspring. His rented farm was in a beautiful setting, overlooking the gentle slopes towards the Yorkshire Wolds. But beautiful views didn't pay the rent and farming was tough for Ivan. He was a tall and silent man, a bit like Frankenstein's monster in both demeanour and appearance, and, during any conversation, the blank expression on his face never changed. The image that sticks in my mind of Ivan is of him trundling around the farm in his little digger. It had a small cabin, not much larger than the farmer himself, with an open front and no windscreen. I think it was called a 'bobcat' and it moved like a tank, with a left and right brake to slow down forward movement on one side or the other. The scoop at the front moved up and down, temporarily obscuring the large face of the slightly maniacal farmer who sat behind it. Ivan grinned or grimaced from the far side of the scoop as he attacked piles of pig manure and scooped it away. Blue fumes issued from the back of the little machine, as it toiled away at Ivan's enthusiastic scooping and scraping. It was the only time he showed any animation.

He was driving in his usual frenzy when I arrived to see a sow with a prolapse. He didn't see me pulling into the yard, and there was no easy way of attracting his attention, so I simply watched his frantic digging as the little buggy rocked and strained against the perpetual mountain of muck. Eventually, I caught his attention and he turned off the noisy engine and squeezed himself out of the tiny cockpit.

Nowadays, commercial pig units are huge and there is almost no individual medicine practised – it is not economic, apparently, to treat an individual pig. A handful of specialist pig vets cover most of the pig farms in the country, advising on feeding regimes and dose rates for antibiotic or minerals to be added to food. They spend more time travelling up and down motorways in air-conditioned cars than they do putting prolapses back into sows. I have not been on a 'proper' commercial pig farm for years, but back in the mid-1990s, in the early years of my veterinary career, there were still some smaller pig herds around and still enough sick pigs to add to the rich variety of work in a mixed veterinary practice. In those days, the indelible smell of a pig was never far away.

Ivan was concerned about his sow. If her prolapse was not corrected, she wouldn't survive, much less give birth to another litter.

'She's got a prolapse. She's over here,' he said, slowly and succinctly. Ivan used as few words as he could get away with, each of them uttered very slowly, as if to use too many or to talk more quickly was a strain on his brain.

'What sort of prolapse is it, Ivan?' I asked. Prolapses could be vaginal or rectal and pre- or post-partum. While the procedure for treating them is basically similar, the likelihood of success varies greatly.

'It's out of its arse,' he replied, bluntly.

I knew exactly what Ivan meant: this was a rectal prolapse, where part of the rectal mucous membrane bulges out, everting through the anus. This is an interesting problem and is seen in pigs for various reasons. Commonly, a young, growing pig might develop a rectal prolapse during a bout of diarrhoea, where straining and inflammation of the lower bowel causes the anal sphincter to give way. It's sometimes also seen in growing pigs if they develop respiratory disease; a chronic cough can lead to bouts of increased intra-abdominal pressure, forcing the rectum to burst out. Similar pressure changes happen if a dairy cow coughs. The health consequences are less, but there is a lot more mess. Semi-solid faeces are forced out under the high pressure generated by the cough and can travel a surprisingly long way. This is why you should never stand behind a coughing dairy cow.

Growing pigs are usually housed in large straw yards with twenty or more unruly adolescents together, and in these cases a prolapsed rectum is an extremely bad thing. The everted, swollen tissue – the shape of an aubergine but the colour of a tomato – is quickly traumatised by the other pigs. Either the affected pig dies, or the prolapse drops off and a rectal stricture forms, rendering it difficult for the pig to pass faeces. Surprisingly, if the pig escapes death, it usually copes quite well, despite its compromised backside. In years gone by, farm animal vets would treat hundreds of pigs like this every year. Nowadays, because of economics, I reckon a pig vet would hardly ever treat such a case.

But Ivan's patient was not a growing pig. She was a sow and heavily pregnant. The pressure inside her belly, as a result of a long uterus full of piglets and fluid, had increased to the point where something had to give. She wasn't quite due to farrow so, at this time, the point of greatest weakness was her anus. It had given way.

Ivan and I stared at the back end of the sow. She seemed remarkably unperturbed by the problem. I'd seen lots of cases like this in ewes just before lambing, where a distended rumen is enough to push things out of the normal boundaries of the body. Pigs do not have a rumen – their digestive system is very similar to a human's – and so pre-partum rectal prolapses are relatively rare. This was the first one I'd seen and I pondered how to tackle it.

'Can you fix her?' asked Ivan, slowly, rubbing his forehead as if to emphasise the depth of his thought process.

'I think so,' I replied, cautiously. 'I'll give her an epidural injection first, then push it back in and put a purse-string suture around.'

I had never given a pig an epidural injection before, but it was essential to relax and numb the area so she wouldn't keep pushing the prolapse back out as I tried to replace it. I assumed that it couldn't be that different from giving an epidural in any other animal, although I racked my brains to remember the depth of the epidural space in a pig's lumbar and sacral spine. I rubbed my forehead like Ivan, trying to hide my true anxieties about the possible outcome.

'I want you to fix her,' Ivan almost pleaded. 'She's worth a bit and she's due to farrow soon, so it's her babies I'm worried about too. Try to save her if you can, please. I know it'll cost me, but I can't deal with any more losses, you know?'

For a tenant farmer like Ivan, making a living by farming pigs was a huge challenge. Wild swings in the pig market resulted in massive fluctuations in the financial viability of the farm, but these were fluctuations over which the farmer had no control. Tenants had to continue to pay the rent, buy feed and clear the vet bills every month, even though the price they received for the finished pig would sometimes be less than the amount it had cost to rear them. If prices were good there was a slight profit, but when the price of bacon or pork plummeted, then the resultant debts could become overwhelming. Economies of scale could mitigate some of the risk, but this did not apply to Ivan, whose farm was quite small.

Despite his quiet exterior, Ivan's anxieties were very real and I suspected his vigorous digger action provided at least something of an outlet for some of his frustration. The rubbing of his forehead was a sign of his ongoing anguish. I sympathised, but I knew the cost of treating his sow would not amount to more than twenty or thirty pounds. Perhaps my use of words like 'epidural' and 'purse-string suture' had set alarm bells ringing that this would be a complicated and hugely expensive procedure. As I gathered my equipment, I tried to reassure Ivan that this would not be the case.

I chose the longest and thinnest needle I could find and

attached it to my small syringe of local anaesthetic, then felt carefully for the landmarks I needed to administer the epidural. Having swabbed the area with surgical spirit, I inserted the needle full-length into the pig's spinal cord, just above her curly tail. It had to go right in the centre. The coil of her tail made it hard to judge exactly the correct position, but I hoped for the best, knowing I'd never be able to replace the prolapse if this didn't work. There was a bit of squealing, but it was no worse than when any pig is injected with a needle. I felt a surge of adrenalin as I depressed the plunger on the syringe. Would it work? Would the sow be paralysed for ever? I was soon to find out, as I withdrew the needle and finally exhaled. Ivan, just as worried but for different reasons, kept on rubbing his forehead and I waited for the signs of epidural success. To my relief, the curly tail went floppy almost immediately – a sure sign that the injection had worked. It also went straight. This was the first success. Ivan was still worried, because to him the problem still looked the same – the huge, red, swollen rectal mass was still there – but for me the hardest part was done. Replacing the everted rectum should be straightforward. Some lubricant and gentle manipulation worked a treat and it quickly disappeared whence it came, with a satisfying plop.

The relief on the farmer's face was as immediate as the relief to the sow. I could see Ivan's mood lift, the strain dissipating from the furrows on his face. I hadn't quite finished, because I needed to place a neat, circular suture around the distorted anus to keep the rectum in place until the swelling went down and the straining stopped, but we both knew the worst was over. Ivan relaxed and started to talk in sentences of more than just the bare minimum of words. As I carefully manoeuvred my needle to make the purse-string, I asked him about his farm and his family. The farm was ticking along, he explained.

'It's just about breaking even, which is better than a lot of pig farms these days.'

On the topic of his family, Ivan was effusive. His son had just completed part of a project in woodwork, and he waxed lyrical about the ingenuity and practicality of what he had made – a device that solved a serious problem in the Stubbs household.

'He's made a thing that holds bottles of brown sauce upside down, so you can get the last bit out. He's a good lad and once he's finished school he's gonna come and help me on the farm,' Ivan declared, bursting with pride.

With the invention of the inverted bottle-holder, I could tell that teatimes in the Stubbs household would be much happier. As I placed the last suture and tied the knot, I was just as delighted there was one less porcine problem too!

I washed off and cleaned up and waved Ivan goodbye. There was less stress on his face. Was that even a smile? I'd saved his pig but who could tell whether it had saved his bacon?

At the other end of the pig farming scale was a farmer I found myself sitting beside at an agricultural society dinner. He owned a huge pig herd as part of his large estate. In the days when there was money to be made from pigs, he had obviously made plenty, because his hobby was collecting art. He recounted to me the story of how this love of art had started, back in the nineties.

The band Blur were playing at a music festival nearby, and were looking for a building on which they could have a promotional piece of graffiti art painted. His pig buildings, by serendipitous chance, happened to be right next door to the estate on which the music festival took place, and he agreed that the band could use one of the buildings as a canvas for the promotional piece. The mural was painted on one side of a breezeblock wall and a rickety wooden door. On the other side were the pigs. The band members were duly photographed in front of the graffiti, although the artist himself furiously avoided being photographed and slipped away, broadly unnoticed. The caravan of publicity moved on. Some months later, the building needed to be modernised and the wall needed to be knocked down. The farmer's daughter asked if she could keep part of the door with the artist's work on. To cut a long story short, the tatty piece of rough wooden door was subsequently sold at auction for tens of thousands of pounds. The artist, it turned out, was Banksy. The rest of the demolished block work was retrieved and also taken to auction. It was sold as one of the most expensive bits of breezeblock from a pig farm ever.

As the dinner went on, I learnt more about his art collection and his life and interests beyond pigs. He reminded me of a pig farmer who I knew at the outset of my career, called Bill. In the days when wealthy, land-owning farmers had a diverse portfolio of animals and crops, pigs were usually part of a big farm's enterprise. The combination of youthful enthusiasm on my part and the healthy price of pigs meant that I often had the freedom to tackle challenges that would have been out of the question on Ivan's farm.

I remembered once being called by Bill to help a farrowing sow. I left the practice before lunch, for what should have been a simple job. If the problem piglet is within arm's reach (not always a foregone conclusion because a pig's uterus is very long), then the slippery little creature, somewhat like a wet bar of soap, can be coaxed out. If not, oxytocin is injected. This is a natural hormone that causes the uterus to contract and expel the unborn piglet. In other species, there can be all sorts of complications in the birth process, leading to difficulties called dystocia. Foetal size, mal-presentation or jumbled-up babies mean strenuous and skilful manipulations are usually required to deal with dystocia.

If these fail, then a Caesarean section is required. But with pigs, where piglets – which are very small in comparison to the sow, and which don't have long, gangly legs to tangle up – shoot alternately along the two long uterine horns, it's a matter of either reach-in-and-pull-it-out, or let-the-drugs-do-the-work. No vet or farmer in their right mind would contemplate a Caesarean on a pig.

When I arrived on Bill's farm, he took me to the patient, who was lying in a farrowing pen. She had been in labour for some time, but no piglets had been forthcoming. I quickly realised I had a problem. I could feel no piglets at all, even with my arm reaching in right up to my armpit. Bill had already given multiple doses of oxytocin, without any success. I looked at Bill and Bill looked at me and we both wondered what to do. Without quite engaging my brain to my mouth, I heard myself declare, 'The only thing I can possibly do to help is to perform an emergency Caesarean section.' I knew the implications of this. I knew Bill would give the green light – money was no object and he always wanted to do the best for his animals. I would be about to tackle an incredibly difficult procedure for the first time on a very challenging patient. I gathered my nerves, my composure and my equipment.

So, why is it so hard (or so foolhardy) to perform a Caesarean section on a pig? It can be done with relative ease on other animals, after all. Well, pigs vehemently dislike injections of any type, so instilling the local anaesthetic to numb the lower flank is difficult. And the sow needs to be sedated. A full general anaesthetic is possible on a small, pet pig, but not on a farm on a huge, pink commercial breed like a Landrace. Even if sedated, the pig is hard to restrain properly and the intestines are prone to escaping through the low flank incision. In addition to this, the two uterine horns are unfeasibly long, so recovering the piglets is like massaging clementines down the longest ever Christmas stocking. In short, it's not simple. The only thing making this surgery easier than it would be on any other animal was the lack of hair. At least I didn't need to clip my patient! Nowadays, YouTube has videos of how to do everything from mending a puncture to complex surgical procedures, but back in the nineties I had to crack on using what I already knew and extrapolating from previous experience.

The veterinary textbook *Techniques in Large Animal Surgery* typically understates the challenges of this procedure, although it does concede that there are some for what it describes as the 'neophyte surgeon'. I certainly fitted the bill for being a 'neophyte' and, as I made my preparations, I took another deep breath. The early part of my veterinary career seemed to be full of deep breaths.

I pressed on nevertheless. I found the uterus more easily than I had expected and made my first cut into it to expose a piglet. More followed as I pushed my arm into the never-ending uterus as if I was donning a thick woollen jumper. I closed one hole and made another, pulling out more and more slimy little piglets, like a fisherman on a spree. At last I thought I was done, but could I be certain there were no more piglets inside? I delved deeper for a final check, my arm surrounded by intestines. The uterus was empty and I started to close up.

Meanwhile, Bill was beaming. His confidence in our joint decision to embark on such a challenging on-farm surgery seemed to have paid off. He had a pile of healthy piglets, which were starting to get in my way. As I carefully sutured back together all the layers of abdominal muscle and skin, the little piglets scurried around my knees, looking for teats. It looked as if mum was going to make it through. It was a great credit to Bill that he had given this 'neophyte' a chance to save the sow and her piglets. He was neither concerned about the cost of the operation, which would run to a small fortune, nor the huge tract of time it had taken me. I shuddered to think what the bill would amount to, but this was the least of my worries now. I had to get back to the practice to help with evening surgery. My absence must have surely been noted – I should only have been away for twenty minutes or so, and that had been four hours ago!

And noted my absence certainly was! My boss was red-faced and furious. He must have presumed I'd fallen asleep after my lunch, or made an alternative appointment rather than help get through the queue of sick dogs and poorly cats queuing in the waiting room.

'Where the *heck* do you think you've been?' he bellowed as he shuffled past me, stooped, stressed and hassled. 'Afternoon surgery has been *really* busy and we've been short-staffed! That pig should not have taken more than twenty minutes! How long does it take to inject a dose of oxytocin, for Christ's sake?'

'Sorry I'm late,' was all I could mutter by way of apology. But then, without a trace of triumphalism (I think) I added, 'I've just been doing a Caesarean on a pig.' I stuck my head out into the waiting room to call in a patient, 'Mrs Harrison and Tiggy? Would you like to come through?'

As Tiggy came into my consulting room, I caught a glimpse of the furious face of my boss, which had immediately changed. The steam from his ears dissipated and the angrily dilated pupils had narrowed. His mouth fell open.

'You've done a Caesarean on a pig?'

Beetroot Sandwiches

When I was a veterinary student, one of the first farms on which I worked was a pig farm. It belonged to two brothers who were sure, one day, to attain the status of farmers who drove large vehicles with small number plates and didn't smell all the time. At this stage though, they were focusing all their efforts on the hard-work phase of their farming lives. The farm was close to my home in Castleford and every day I would cycle there, with my wellies and sandwiches in a rucksack, to help out and learn as much as I could about pigs. On my first day, I was shown the computer program used for optimising production, to allow maximum growth of weaned pigs at a minimal cost. Spreadsheets held no interest for me and I had to stifle my yawns. I just wanted to get on with looking after the animals.

The next day, I was let loose on the pigs. At first, I had simple jobs like feeding the newly purchased gilts (young female pigs). They were kept in confinement for a few weeks, partly to ensure they didn't have any disease, but also because they needed to be housed away from the males until such time as they appeared to be coming into season. This was another job of mine, even at this early stage of my animal husbandry career – to check if any of the gilts under my care were coming into heat. I had to push down on their backs, to mimic the weight of a boar during the mating process. If they stood still, then this was a sign of impending oestrus. I also had to observe their vulvas twice every day for signs of swelling. As a teenage boy, this messed with my mind somewhat, but before long I was an expert.

There was a lot to learn and the whole experience of being on a pig farm was filled with new stimuli to all the senses. Pigs make the most interesting noises, from the contented grunts of a happy pig, snuffling and rooting its bedding or in a pile of mud, to the high-pitched squeals and melodramatic shrieks when things don't go according to the pig's plan. Some pig farmers, apparently, like to wear ear defenders to protect their ears from that particular noise. And as for the smells! Pig farms have a distinct odour, which is very different from other types of farm. There are none of the fruity, esterified organic molecules from silage that typify the fragrance of a herd of cows, nor the warm, comforting smell of lanolin that is synonymous with sheep. Instead there is a dryer, flatter and more acrid smell with notes of ammonia. As I was to learn very quickly, the smell of pigs has pervasive and indelible characteristics, which penetrate protective clothing and even the pores of the skin.

Since I was a student, and always in need of funds, I had managed, alongside my stints at the pig farm, to pin down an evening job at a local pizza takeaway. It had the unlikely name of Tudor Cottage, presumably due to the faux black and white exterior of the converted bookmakers shop in which it had been recently opened. It occurred to me that the name was entirely unsuitable, because pizza would certainly not have been on the menu in

Tudor Britain. It probably hadn't even been invented in Italy at the time of Henry VII! Regardless of the name, the appearance of a pizza takeaway in Castleford was cause for excitement. It made a change from the traditional and ubiquitous fish and chips. Soon after Tudor Cottage opened, my dad started a habit that would stay with me for several decades – and counting – of having pizza on a Saturday night for tea. On that first occasion, he walked down the road to collect our order of garlic bread, a safe ham and mushroom pizza and a more exotic new variety called a Chin Dripper. It was number ten on the list. For some reason, this is forever etched on my mind. My dad, like lots of people in Castleford at this time, was not used to collecting and carrying flat, square boxes of pizza and he tucked them under his arm in just the same way as he would carry a newspaper from the newsagent's next door. Needless to say, by the time he arrived home to the Norton family, who were eagerly awaiting their new and exciting takeaway, all the Chin Dripper topping had slid off the pizza, leaving a naked circle of dough and a sloppy pile of topping soaked into the corner of the box. Our first pizza was not a great success. The following day, however, I called in to Tudor Cottage and asked for a job. I think the new owners reasoned that my family's weekly purchases would cover my meagre wages, which were just two pounds an hour. I started work there the following week.

What the owners didn't know, and what I didn't yet know either, was that working on a pig farm by day and taking money and adding pepperoni to deep pan pizzas by evening was not an ideal combination. The two-hour gap between one job and the other was utterly inadequate to remove the all-pervading smell of pig, which exuded from every inch of my skin. I scrubbed my way through bars and bars of yellow, coal tar soap, which, according to consensus, was the cleanser of choice for removing pig smell. The combination of pig farm and tar soap did not go perfectly with pizzas, however. The owners were too polite to comment, but I am sure my odiferous presence in front of house and at the pizza oven was one of the reasons the business never took off.

But, back at the farm, I was getting used to the smell and gleaning as much as I could about pigs. I was hungry for knowledge and I hoped that the pig man, whose name was Iggy, would help. He surely had a wealth of information about everything to do with pigs. On occasions, talking to himself in incoherent grunts, he even sounded like one!

Whether Iggy was his actual name I never knew. The only other Iggy I had heard of had the surname 'Pop'. Pig man Iggy had only one characteristic in common with Iggy Pop, and that was his wizened and wiry physique. Pig man Iggy was not flamboyant and did not sing songs. Pig man Iggy also had a bulbous nose, bent to one side of his face, and a shuffling, mildly uncoordinated gait. If he ever moved quickly, his shuffling uncoordination made it likely that he'd fall over, so he usually moved quite slowly. Luckily, he was nearly always pushing a wheelbarrow, which gave him extra stability. He was short and completely bald with a round and pink head, somewhat like the creatures he was looking after. He would have been a great source of knowledge, had I ever managed to maintain a proper conversation with him. Goodness knows I tried enough times, but he didn't want to engage in any type of conversation about pigs and when he did talk to me, the words came out of his mouth in a sort of grunting snort, so it was hard to understand anything he said anyway.

While I undertook my daily tasks on the farm, dished out by the boss, Iggy was busy with his usual work, wheeling manure, removing dead piglets to the muck heap and so on. He was too busy to talk. On most days, I was also too busy to talk, because I would have been given a list of jobs of gargantuan proportions by the farmer.

Once, with a glint in one eye and his other eye on the spreadsheet of costs, he handed me a syringe, a handful of needles and a couple of large, plastic bottles containing life-preserving vaccine.

'Today's job, Julian, is to vaccinate all these sows,' he explained, waving his arm as if to display his herd. Mercifully, he demonstrated how to do this, on one sow; but only one. Then he left me to it, for me to learn as I went. I gazed across the huge straw yard, full of sows, as ovoid as zeppelins as they sauntered around the building. It was a peaceful place, full of about two hundred pregnant sows. Peaceful, at least, until I appeared with my clumsy needle and novice technique. Every single pig, resting or calmly rooting in the straw, squealed (like a pig) with surprise and objection when I stabbed my needle into her neck.

A few years later, during the clinical part of our training at Cambridge Vet School, our senior lecturer in large animal medicine, Dr Jackson, gave us some advice.

'The thing with pigs,' he counselled, 'is that you need *stealth*.'

I'd learnt this important lesson in that barn, as big as a football pitch, as I attempted to inject several hundred pigs in just one day. What Dr Jackson didn't say was that the other key ingredient was *speed*. A combination of stealth and speed gave me half a chance of completing the task. After a couple of hours, with several doses of vaccine squirted, by accident, into the floppy ears of the intended recipients, I'd got the knack. I'd stealthily sneak up on a sleeping sow and jab her in the neck, just behind the ear. If I was quick and I could keep close to the patient, I'd be able to depress the plunger and deliver the dose of vaccine. If she threw her head up, or ran away too quickly, or tried to sink her teeth into my leg, then the dose was wasted, throwing the spreadsheet of costings into disarray and usually throwing me into the straw. The following day I had another set of jabs to give and before long I was fully competent at injecting pigs – a skill that has stayed with me to this day!

There was a brief hiatus in my pig handling, when I was given the job of spraying every slat and slurry surface with some noxious chemical to kill flies. I had to dress up in a bright green plastic suit with a hood, which made me look a bit like one of Robin Hood's friends. It was also very hot and sweaty, partly because it was a plastic suit and partly because pigs inside a low-ceilinged building generate a lot of heat. And as they are not hairy or woolly, pigs' body heat is not trapped next to their skin and instead leaves their body and warms up everything nearby. I was given a small bottle of concentrated solution, which had yellow warning triangles with pictures of dead fish on its label. I poured it, as instructed, into a pressurised sprayer, like those used to kill greenfly on roses, and then topped it up with water from the hosepipe.

Spraying this stuff in all the smelliest parts of the farm was my least favourite job. I had to constantly wipe my forehead. It was hard to know whether it was the heat of the plastic suit or the powerful chemical fumes that made my body wet and my eyes sting. I'd never find out, because next I was moved back to an animal-related task. Thank goodness.

Once I'd mastered the toxic third role, I was fast-tracked to the inseminating shed, where the sows were lined up with their swollen vulvas pointing towards the alleyway, along which I prowled like a seedy stalker. Some lucky sows would be corralled into the boar pen, where they would be mated by an actual pig. I could never understand how it was decided which sows had that luxury while others could only look forward to a thin plastic tube when they were in season. I watched the boars in action, first sniffing, then mounting their partner in a process that could last as long as fifteen minutes. The farmer would often supervise – mainly to make sure everything went where it was supposed to go. This was clearly important in any animal, but especially with an inexperienced pig. The volume of ejaculate was huge and could easily fill a milk bottle. If the boar was clumsy or the farmer was not quick to intervene, much of this fluid could end up squirting down the farmer's wellie, with the obvious unwanted results of no pregnancy and wet socks. I never progressed to the heady heights of supervising the mating, but I was pleased to be back in hands-on animal action. My job in this shed was to administer an altogether different injection to the vaccinations of the sow house. I had to inject semen! It came in a plastic bottle – like the ones containing the white not-so-sticky-glue that young children use at school – and it needed to be squirted down a plastic tube into each sow in the optimistic hope that it would end up somewhere in the proximity of an ovulating ovary. On my first day of this job, the boss was off again – he had a meeting with a feed supplier – and Iggy was busy with his favourite job of shovelling dead piglets into the muck heap. The responsibility for fathering a whole generation of piglets on the farm fell to me. I had been shown what to do, but just once, so once again I had to learn quickly.

A sow's cervix, through which the semen needs to be squirted, is threaded, like a nut and bolt. The long, bendy plastic catheter is designed with a matching thread and so, once lubricated and inserted, needs to be turned, anticlockwise like the thread of a Calor gas connector, before the semen is instilled. To be fair, it was simpler than it sounded, but my biggest issue was the lack of any sort of introduction. I'd just appear behind the poor sow, kneel down, pull the top off the bottle, lube my catheter, insert, twist, then squeeze. A degree of pressure was needed, but some of the sows would seem to 'drink the semen' and the contents of the bottle would disappear without the need to squeeze at all. I wanted to discuss this phenomenon with someone who knew, and I resolved to pluck up the courage to ask Iggy next time we were together and he wasn't shovelling dead piglets. There were questions for which I needed answers. How many piglets did each sow produce? (The answer seemed to be multiple.) And how many teats did each sow have anyway? (The answer to this seemed to be not quite enough – pig breeders were busy engineering sows to be long, with more udder space to accommodate the exponential production of piglets at this time.) For now, I'd be content with an explanation of what I'd just seen with the bottle of semen. After each insemination, I scribbled the date and time on the little blackboard behind each sow, like notching up conquests on the headboard of a busy bed in a bordello.

My chance to ask Iggy my burning question was during the 'snap' break – the time allotted in the middle of the day to eat sandwiches. We would congregate in a tiny room, which contained a fridge, a kettle and a table and chairs. Iggy only ever drank diluted orange squash and only ever ate beetroot sandwiches, a habit that I too acquired over the time I was with him. Every time I eat a beetroot sandwich now I think of Iggy, his bent nose and his grunting voice. For some reason, it never puts me off my lunch.

While the pig man fitted the squash bottle under his bent nose, I plucked up courage to ask his advice about the phenomenon of semen sucking. I described what I'd seen several times that morning, which I thought was fascinating. I thought maybe I had discovered something new.

'Could this actually happen, Iggy?' I asked, describing how the sows seemed to drink the semen. After Iggy had digested the final bite of his beetroot sandwich and washed it down with squash, he answered my question, succinctly, before standing up to return to his wheelbarrow.

'Aye,' he said. Followed by a grunt. Then he was off to find dead piglets.

During that month-long placement, I learnt a lot about pigs. How to inject them, how to check if they were in season and even how to inseminate them. It had been a good summer. But all I gained from Iggy was a love of beetroot sandwiches.

Has Anyone Seen our Sow?

The stone farmhouse at the end of the tree-lined drive was imposing. Draped in wisteria, which enveloped the whole house with cascading purple blossom, it should have been one of the most beautiful buildings in the most beautiful part of Yorkshire. But there was an element of tatty neglect. The Yorkshire stone, so common in all the surrounding villages, usually shone with a rich, golden hue, but here it was gloomy and had a greyish tinge, overshadowed as it was by enormous trees. I paused halfway up the drive to try to weigh up the place and get a sense of what might be in store. There were cattle to the left, with shaggy coats and huge horns. A couple of pigs rooted in the muddy field to the right, adjacent to a small wood, and chickens pecked about in the spaces between. I had been invited for lunch and I was struggling to fathom why.

I had recently started work in the practice and I was beginning to become familiar with some of the farming fraternity. I had met the owners of this organic farm just once, briefly and in passing outside the practice. They were depositing a faeces sample and I simply took the plastic pot off their hands. As well as the pot, I took their names, the name of their farm, what the sample was and what needed to be tested. I didn't think I'd made such an impression that an invitation to lunch was warranted.

Of course, I'd made a few enquiries prior to accepting. The local farming community is always a great source of information and I'd found out some facts. Viola and Sebastian had a small farm. Their farm was extensive, with almost zero intervention from the farmers. It ticked all the boxes in the organic farming rulebook. Indeed, some said they had written the rulebook. Just like on George Orwell's Manor Farm, all animals on this farm were equal and free to roam where they pleased and eat what they wished. The paradigm of socialist equality extended to Viola and Sebastian's own ideology and, according to local gossip, their socialist principles were as strong as those of the leaders parodied by Orwell. I expected my lunch date would be an interesting experience. I wondered whether the farming couple had invited all new vets to their farm – I could not see how I justified a special invitation.

I stood at the door and rang the bell, feeling moderately uncomfortable. Shortly, Viola arrived, dressed in a tweed skirt and a headscarf. She had obviously dressed up for the occasion. The pile of mud-covered wellies, sticks, coats, overalls and hats that took up much of the entrance hall told me that the usual attire was typical farmwear.

'Do come in, Julian. It's so nice of you to join us,' she effused, in an accent not dissimilar to that of Tricki Woo's owner from the famous James Herriot stories. 'We're having gin and tonic, would you like one?'

I politely declined, accepting just a tonic. At some point later, I had to go back to work. There was a farm visit with my name against it and also evening surgery to complete, so my sojourn needed to be fairly brief. If the worst came to the worst, at least I had an excuse to get away. Lunchtime drinking, at least for this veterinary surgeon in the 1990s, was off the cards. Once upon a time, though, any equine vet worth his salt would have accepted the gin, followed it with wine, then settled in with whisky to watch the afternoon racing on the telly.

Before having lunch, we sat at either side of the enormous drawing room. They both seemed very interested to hear about my background and quizzed me about what it was like to have been brought up in industrial West Yorkshire. I think they must have thought I had actually worked down a coal mine, because I quickly reached the conclusion that they had labelled me as their token 'working-class' friend. I felt like Sean Bean when he played the gruff gardener in the TV adaptation of *Lady Chatterley*. I sipped at my tonic with increasing nervousness.

Lunch followed, equally spread out because the dining room was massive and so was the table at which we sat. I almost had to shout to make myself heard. While spooning pea and ham soup, I asked about the farm – how many and what sort of animals they looked after. All farmers love to talk about their animals, so this part of the conversation was easier. I was pleased to have moved on from the interrogation regarding my perceived working-class roots (I don't think my background and upbringing was quite what they had hoped for). They spoke with passion about their organic aspirations, but it was hard to agree with some of their ideas.

'We don't use any wormers or anything like that, do we Sebastian?' declared Viola. Sebastian nodded, adding, 'and no vaccines, or antibiotics. Everything is natural here!'

It was when the topic of conversation turned to homeopathic medications that I started to fidget uncomfortably. They, apparently, added watery liquids called nosodes into the water troughs that the cattle drank out of, to prevent a variety of illnesses. Without any rationale behind the use of these liquids and, worse, without any evidence of the efficacy (let alone safety – although a small bottle of water is surely very safe), I could not support their vigorous assertions that this constituted best practice. Isolated as I was at the far end of a huge table, I felt hamstrung. I was desperate to argue the case for the tried and tested conventional medication regimes, but it was neither the time nor the place to make a case or provoke an argument. I remained polite and, as such, complicit, the guest that I was intended to be.

'Anyway, you *must* come and look at the animals,' Sebastian urged, to my relief. The soup and bread was finished and now seemed a perfect time to get outside.

'That's a great idea. I'd love to,' I agreed vigorously, 'And thank you so much for the lovely soup. I'll get my wellies.'

The farm tour started in the cow house, which was piled high with a mixture of bedding and manure. The three of us leant on the gate and looked in. At head height, two cows lay, chewing their cud and apparently quite content.

'We run a deep-litter system here,' Sebastian confirmed as I eyed the bedding. At well over a metre deep, it was a very deep-litter system. One that had not been cleared out for several years. So established was the deep bedding that the fungal colonies must have been numerous. I suspected a whole ecosystem flourished beneath its surface.

'But our cows just love to spend time outside in the woods,' Viola added. 'They are free to roam wherever they please, you see.'

We climbed the gate and struggled over the uneven surface, occasionally tripping over hens that were resting in divots, and headed to the fold yard, where I was surprised to see some small sheep loitering over a pile of musty hay.

'Most of the sheep are outside. We prefer it if they lamb in the fresh air,' Sebastian explained.

'How was lambing time?' I asked, always an important question in May. They would surely have just finished the busiest part of the farming year and mothers with strong lambs would be enjoying the late spring weather.

'Well, Julian, to be truthful, lambing time is still happening. We let our rams live with the flock all year round, so lambing is an ongoing thing for us. We get lambs arriving all through summer!' Viola explained, with some pride. I tried not to let my raised eyebrows be too obvious. This was a really bad way to run a flock. Natural as it might be, it is almost impossible to provide proper antenatal care to ewes if nobody knows when they are due to give birth, let alone to provide supervision if the sheep encounters problems at parturition. It would surely be even worse if the expectant mum is somewhere in the middle of the woods!

And it was the woods where we headed next, the main stomping ground of the pigs. Pigs are great creatures and love rooting and rummaging in and amongst trees and undergrowth. It may be that woods constitute the natural home of the pig. Their wild boar ancestors would have thrived in ancient forests, finding beechnuts and maybe even truffles if they were lucky! If you are a modern wild boar living on the tree-covered slopes of mountains in spacious southern France, this is still fine. There are acres of space to root around in, and a French wild boar would be more likely to encounter Ben Fogle exploring life in the wild than find itself sharing a wood with another pig or upturning the same bit of woodland floor over and over again. However, in a small patch of woodland on a ramshackle farm, even just a few pigs quickly trash the delicate arboreal biome. Far from it being a utopian vision of health, with spring flowers sprouting from lush, green grass and bluebells carpeting the forest floor, this was a quagmire, reminiscent of the Somme.

'Our pigs just love it in these woods,' Sebastian explained. I spotted a couple in the distance, covered in mud. One was struggling to extricate itself from the goo. Wholesome and natural as it undoubtedly was, I couldn't help but have my concerns over whether this was altogether the best environment for the pigs to thrive.

'Julian! Look at Harry and Henrietta! Harry's our wonderful boar – he's absolutely wonderful. Henrietta is his best friend. They're always together,' Viola shouted, as she, too, spotted the couple struggling in the distance. To complete the sorry scene, a trail of brown piglets followed behind Henrietta. Periodically, one would fall in a puddle, emerging squeaking and wet moments later. I tried to imagine they were enjoying it – like a rugby player on a wet day rather than an infantryman on the western front. Having just watched a series of unfortunate piglets become completely submerged (they all eventually reappeared), I felt it was time to go. I'd enjoyed the soup and bread, but was not convinced by the farmers' idea of running a healthy farm.

'Viola, Sebastian, it's been really interesting looking around your farm and thank you for lunch. I really should go. I have some blood tests to do later this afternoon, then evening surgery. I don't want to be late,' I said. 'Is there a hosepipe to clean my wellies?' ' I half expected to be shown to the well to get my water. ('It's more natural that way.')

As I tidied up and washed off, Viola gushed, 'It's been lovely to meet you. You should come again. We have so many friends we'd like you to meet!'

I felt this was shaping up for me to be paraded as the token salt-of-the-earth Yorkshire coal-mining man again, so my enthusiasm was muted.

'Anyway, Julian, Sebastian and I wondered if you could help. We've lost our favourite sow, Francesca. She lives in the woods and we haven't seen her for days. We wondered if you could keep an eye out, or let us know if anyone finds a sow? It's probably Francesca. We'd be very grateful if you could put the word about.'

I couldn't help but smile as I drove back down the potholed farm track towards the road. I knew there was zero chance of persuading the pair into a more conventional way of farming. I've met several farmers like this, often son and mother or siblings working together day in, day out. They're close-knit, old-fashioned and, by nature, inward-looking. Suggesting changes or updated methods is, I've come to learn, often fruitless. I hoped they were happy, living the dream of ultimate farming freedom. But I did wonder whether the animals were happy, atop the ceiling-high deep-litter bedding, heaving through gloopy mud or drinking ineffective homeopathic nosodes that would afford them no proper protection against any illness.

Some weeks later, there was a message in the daybook at the practice. Sebastian and Viola had found Francesca, their lost sow. She was dead, squashed under a tree that had come down in a recent storm, in the boggy wood.

To quote George Orwell again, 'All animals are equal but some animals are more equal than others.'

Certainly not Boaring

I was in the midst of morning surgery when my phone pinged. Between consults, I glanced at the message. It was not from a client, but from a friend. Kimry was a vet, and used to work with my wife. She specialised in horses, but had become embroiled in managing other types of animals on a rescue farm. As well as the ponies and donkeys that were Kimry's area of expertise, there were pigs, goats, alpacas and sheep, which also needed to be looked after. While she did have some experience with farm animals, it was pushing her out of her comfort zone, which was where I came in. The contents of the text message were enough to strike fear into the soul of many vets:

Hi Julian! Just a quick question – would you castrate an adult male pig (not massive, one of those Kunekune spotty ones). We've tried the injections to stop his fertility, but it's not been perfect and there's already one litter of unexpected piglets.

As I read and reread the text, I wasn't sure whether the question was asking whether *I* (specifically me) would do the honours on this adult pig, or if *any vet* should attempt to do so. A second message clarified her request:

> Or can you recommend someone? She would like him
> done very shortly as she needs to keep him away from the
> others in the group and he is wrecking the stable.

And then the third added more important information, which suggested it would need more than just one vet:

> I can be there to help you if that would be useful.

It was an ominous prospect. Most vets would have run fast in the opposite direction, wishing to avoid a complicated challenge with an adult boar at all costs. Especially one for a farmer who wasn't even a client of the practice. There was a lot that could go wrong. It would have been easiest to excuse myself as being too busy (which I was), and the farm being too far away (which it also was). However, I liked and admired Kimry. Often over tea or a glass of wine, I'd heard stories of her hard work, enthusiastic endeavours and excellent client care. Recently she had been on maternity leave with her first child and had then started her own independently run, single-handed practice; no mean feat for anyone, let alone a new mother. Her little daughter, apparently, travelled around with her on visits from a very young age.

We had attended the launch party of her new practice, one dark evening at the village hall in East Rounton, a small and typically quaint North Yorkshire village within sight of the North York Moors escarpment. I'd been to the village many times before to treat huge outbreaks of pneumonia in housed cattle on a farm in foggy, damp November. I had spent hours emptying bottles and bottles of medication into calves' veins in an attempt to save their delicate bovine lungs from aggressive respiratory pathogens. We passed the entrance to that farm on the way to Kimry's party. But there was no such gloom at this evening's festivities, just a lot of energy, excitement and plenty of friends to lend their support to her new venture. For nearly two decades now, I'd run a veterinary business, but I had colleagues and partners. Even when working together and pulling hard to make things go smoothly, distributing the work and the responsibilities and sharing the hassles, it was very hard. The negatives of running a small business often overshadowed the positives, especially a small veterinary business, fraught with health and safety issues, regulations and bad debts from ungrateful clients. To be doing it single-handed, taking all the risk on your own and never having an evening without being on call, was something that I could not imagine.

So, despite my deep misgivings about attempting to separate a large pig from his (probably very large) testicles, my response went like this:

Yes, I think I can help. I'll give you a ring tomorrow. What's the best time to call?

I couldn't stop myself from trying to help.

Kimry's reply was simply an emoji with a very smiley face, so I sensed she was pleased to have me shouldering the responsibility of tackling this boar's tackle, so to speak.

Once upon a time, cooperation of this sort was commonplace amongst neighbouring vets. Even back in James Herriot's day, complicated surgery in dogs was referred (or deferred) to Denton

Pette, a vet in Darlington, whose surgical heroism at that time was legendary. Rumour had it that he drove a Bentley, so it is safe to assume that he knew as much about charging for his skills as he did about fixing a broken bone. When I first started working in Thirsk, cases requiring spinal surgery would be sent to a vet called Nigel Harcourt-Brown. He was the Denton Pette of the 1990s.

I remember a Weimaraner dog, called Spookie, who had a rare neurological disease. She needed a spinal tap to analyse the fluid bathing her spinal cord and brain. This was just outside the limits of my novice capability, so I sought the help of Nigel in Harrogate. Nigel performed the tap and sent me a report, complete with lab results, which described and confirmed the condition I suspected – immune mediated meningio-encephalitis – as Spookie's diagnosis. At the bottom of the report, Nigel had commented:

But you'll know much more about how to treat that condition than I do.

He was a senior vet and an expert in his field, but there was nothing patronising about his comments and he was happy to defer to my modern knowledge on immunosuppressive therapy. Some modern-day specialists could learn a lot from the friendly, neighbourly relationships in the veterinary profession's past. Nearly twenty-five years later, as I volunteered to castrate a large adult pig, I hoped I would be as helpful to Kimry as both Nigel and Denton had been in their time.

Castrating an adult boar is not something we do very often. As I drove to the farm, some distance away from the practice but, handily, close to my kids' school (I'd fixed the visit for a day when it was my turn to do the school run), I tried to think back to whether I had done it before. Yes, I had castrated lots of pigs, but they were all either small piglets, in which case the job was simple, or they were pigs of the guinea variety, also reasonably straightforward.

On one occasion, I had a litter of rare-breed piglets to castrate and the owner brought them to the practice in a large wire cage. Six squealing piglets is not a typical thing to see or hear in a vet's waiting room. It was in the early days of filming for *The Yorkshire Vet* and, as usual, I had a camera crew with me, excitedly grabbing anything interesting and hoping for drama. Everyone's interest was piqued and I felt the pressure of expectation again.

Castrating little piglets is really easy. A few millilitres of local into the skin overlying each testicle, one sharp incision followed by steady, constant traction on the testicle to remove it, repeat on the other side and it is done. I completed five of the six piglets in no time. There was no drama to be had, but at least the patients were unusual and very cute. However, what happened on piglet number six was quite unexpected. Unbeknownst to me, the piglet had an inguinal hernia. This is a congenital problem with the small fissure, like a slit, that allows a testicle to descend from the abdomen into the scrotum during the final stages of development in the womb. Usually this closes shortly after birth, when the testicles have dropped, and the abdomen is sealed. But sometimes it stays open, allowing anything else in the abdomen to follow the path of the descended testicle. I cut into and pulled on the piglet's left gonad, only to watch in dismay as all its vermiform intestines followed, spilling out onto the table in front of my very eyes.

I stared at the purple pile, which looked like a bag of snakes, and knew disaster was imminent. I could feel panic rising within me, but tried to remain outwardly calm as I scooped up the unfortunate piglet with its insides out and rushed him to theatre. If I didn't get this fixed quickly, the little pig would die. But luck was on my side and, under quickly induced gaseous anaesthesia, I managed to feed the slippery loops of bowel back into their proper place and suture the hernia closed.

This little piggy had escaped its brush with death. If something similar happened with Kimry's boar, however, it was sure to be a total disaster and one that would guarantee I would never set foot on any of her farms again.

I dropped the kids off at school and headed towards the conspicuous triangle on the horizon that was Roseberry Topping. Kimry's boar was somewhere near the base of this mini-Matterhorn. Roseberry Topping is one of the most distinctive hills in North Yorkshire and towers over the picturesque village of Great Ayton. Until 1912, the summit was shaped like a sugarloaf, but a combination of local mining for both alum and ironstone and the presence of a geological fault caused it to acquire its current vertical western face. Even before its iconic shape was sculpted, Roseberry Topping was a big attraction for climbers.

James Cook, the British explorer, navigator and cartographer who travelled the world, charting known coastlines and discovering others, lived at its base. His ascents of Roseberry Topping, coupled with the expansive views from the summit, seeded his taste for adventure. I pondered whether today's porcine procedure would be similarly epic. Certainly, I couldn't think of any previous occasions when I'd done this on an actual adult pig. I knew it would not be simple – boars are not easy to manage and are difficult to sedate. They also act in a belligerent and often aggressive way towards anyone trying to interfere with their day-to-day business of snuffling and rooting around. Boars have strong necks, big, sharp teeth and can move with surprising speed. Furthermore, they are difficult to restrain adequately, so the task of dealing with them is altogether more challenging than it is in other domestic animals. Horses, even if uncooperative, are used to being handled. Cattle, even if not used to being handled, can be corralled into a cattle crush, which keeps them safe and stationary. Pigs don't fit into either of these categories. They also lack the susceptibility to be persuaded or coerced.

When I arrived, Kimry introduced me to the pig in the stable, who was called Versace, and his owner, who was called Christina. Christina shook my hand and Versace waddled across the stable to say hello. The pig was about the length of a Great Dane dog, but with shorter, stocky legs. Both owner and pig were very friendly. That is, until I tried gently to palpate Versace's testicles. The boar squealed a vigorous objection, opening his jaws and flinging his head around, showering me with saliva and baring his teeth and tusks. The curved weapons narrowly missed my arm and I quickly retreated to make a plan and lick my imagined wounds.

Versace would need sedation of some sort. There is a classic pig sedative called Stressnil. As its name suggests, the purpose is to remove any trace of stress from a pig. However, when faced with an assailant such as a scalpel-wielding vet intent on removing testicles, even a huge dose of this stress-relieving drug has a limited effect. Other sedative drugs commonly used in other species do not seem to work very well in pigs, but there was one horse drug that I knew was helpful if used as part of a combination. Luckily, Kimry had a bottle of this elixir in her car. I made some calculations and mixed up the drugs in a syringe, adding a bit more just for good measure. The syringe was huge and I recalculated my doses several times just to be safe, before skulking back into the pig pen armed with the sedative and a makeshift pig board, adapted from a piece of wooden shelf. Pig boards are useful for herding pigs, or at least offering temporary restraint.

It worked wonders and the two-vet combo had Versace injected slickly and smoothly before he realised what was happening. Now we had to wait. It was time for a coffee and a chat, all the time keeping watch over the stable door to check on the state of Versace's slumber.

We covered lots of topics – how Kimry's practice was developing came up first. She was busy and it was going well: hard work – every night on call was tough (for once, I felt glad of my one-in-two rota), although she cheerfully confirmed that nocturnal disturbance was very rare, at which point I felt imme-diately envious. Christina talked about her animals too, pointing out Amadeus and Ludwig, two alpacas, in the distance, and Versace's recent (accidental) girlfriends and his (unplanned) offspring in the nearby paddock.

'Well, after today there certainly shouldn't be any more unwanted piglets, Christina,' I quipped. She'd tried to keep him separate from the sows, but he kept escaping. Kimry had used injections to try to reduce Versace's libido, again without success. It was a case of either rehoming him to another farm or castrating him, obviously a more permanent solution. Full of hassle as today would be, it seemed the only sensible way to save Versace's bacon.

By the time we'd finished our coffee, it looked as if the drugs had worked. Versace had stopped rooting around his stable and was snoring loudly in the corner. Kimry and I crept in, armed with local anaesthetic – that still needed to be injected into the skin of his scrotum – antiseptic, scalpel and surgical kit. 'What could possibly go wrong?' I thought, putting out of my mind recollections of the piglet whose intestines had unexpectedly fallen out and the saliva-strewn assault from fifteen minutes previously.

With a small-bore needle (a needle of small diameter, I mean, not necessarily one for a small boar), I drew up the local anaesthetic. This is essential because, even though it stings initially, it renders the whole area numb, making the surgery feasible. But as soon as I'd inserted it under his skin, Versace roared into life like a lawnmower and ran off. At least there was no attempt to attack this time. He soon lay back down, this time under a pile of straw, as if trying to hide. 'Seconds out, round two,' I imagined in my head as we went in again. Several years ago, I had a very close shave with a belligerent pig called Monica. She was so aggressive, fiercely protecting her babies, that it was only possible to inject her using a syringe on a long pole. At least Versace was vaguely sedated.

Kimry put a towel over his head and this time managed to pin him down. He needed to stay still long enough for me to give my injection and for his skin to become numb. It worked a treat and, with only minimal objection this time round, the worst part was done. Next I opened the kit, cleaned the area, cleaned my hands and then I was ready to go. One deft slice through the skin exposed the testicle. I extruded it completely – my word, they were big – then applied the emasculators. These are medieval-looking things, somewhat like a pair of secateurs for trimming a rose bush. They both cut and clamp at the same time and, as long as they are applied correctly, 'nut to nut', they do exactly as their name suggests – deprive a male of his masculinity. First one part of Versace's masculine identity was lying in the straw, swiftly followed by the second. The job was done, in the end without even a sniff or grunt of objection. There was no sedative problem, no prolapsed intestines and no injury to the vets. As Kimry went to her car boot to retrieve some spray to apply to the wounds, there was a palpable lifting of tension.

Kimry's topical antimicrobial of choice was a new and fancy spray, made of and also the colour of silver. It was, apparently, all the rage in the equine world. This was very different from the blue spray that was the workhorse of a cattle vet. She passed it to me to apply the finishing touches to the scrotal wounds. I couldn't help but step back to admire the silvery scrotum, now pleasantly devoid of its contents. As Versace snoozed and the three humans breathed a collective sigh of relief, a mischievous thought entered my head. Before I knew what I'd done, Versace had silver trotters to match his silver scrotum – like his namesake, he was the very epitome of fashion.

4. Horses and Donkeys

Had things worked out differently, I might have been a horse vet. Not because I possessed any particular aptitude for the species, nor because I was fascinated by the horse any more than I was any other animal, but purely as a result of geography. Cambridge Vet School, where I did my six years of training to become a veterinary surgeon, was just a few furlongs from Newmarket Heath, the home of flat racing. Newmarket was, and still is, synonymous with all things racehorse and the veterinary practices there are second to none. Rossdales and Greenwood Ellis are possibly two of the most known and respected veterinary practices in the world. As students we used to visit Newmarket periodically, as much to imbibe its history as to learn any specific equine facts. It was an amazing place and, even if you happened to harbour a vigorous dislike for horses (as some did), it was impossible not to be captivated. More recently, I have got to know Peter Rossdale, who established the eponymous equine practice. Now in his nineties, he still goes into the clinic most days. He is one of the great names in modern veterinary work and it is impossible not to become enthralled and inspired by everything equine when in conversation with him.

Then I moved to Thirsk, also in an area with a keen racing heritage. We are surrounded by racecourses – Thirsk, Ripon, Catterick, Wetherby and, of course, York. Hambleton, a small hamlet on the top of Sutton Bank, three hundred metres above sea level, claims to be the 'Home of the Thoroughbred'. Once upon a time, the racecourse here was regarded as one of the finest in the country, second only in importance to Newmarket. In the seventeenth and eighteenth centuries, Hambleton held the most significant race meetings in Yorkshire, including the prestigious Royal Gold Cup. The sloping grassland is still there, and is used as training gallops by trainers Kevin Ryan and Bryan Smart. The weather is usually inclement and, if the wind is from the east, it's freezing. It is hard to imagine the large crowd that would have gathered in 1612, the first recorded date for racing in Hambleton. The unlikely meeting place might have found favour because it is situated right on the old drovers' road, which runs north to south. It would have been a major thoroughfare back then.

Next, I spent a year working in the Cotswolds, just outside Cheltenham. I would see the famous racecourse every day, either in passing or in the distance as I walked the dog on nearby Cleeve Hill. Anne and I worked in a local mixed practice and lived in a tiny, rose-covered cottage in the historic town of Winchcombe. During this time, attempting to fill the boots of the retiring senior vet, I was thrown feet first into equine practice. It was tough. I did my best but, without the correct wellies (mine were farm wellies and not the horsey type) or the full vocabulary of equine terminology, I was always going to struggle to fit in with the horsey crowd. Nevertheless, the infectious enthusiasm of everyone who descended on Winchcombe every March for the Cheltenham Festival was hard to avoid. Every pub, restaurant and hotel overflowed with racegoers, every spare bed for miles around booked up months if not years in advance. It was a week-long party. Usually, I can't help but become embroiled in anything where there is so much unfettered passion, but for some reason I never became as hooked by the horse bug as I might have. Despite that, I still hope that just some of the combined equine heritage of Newmarket, Cheltenham and Hambleton might have rubbed off on me!

Blossom the Shire Horse and Basil the Donkey

Castleford in the 1970s was the epitome of industrial West Yorkshire and hardly the place to spawn a successful veterinary career. Coal mining was still prevalent. Dirty, smoggy industry was everywhere. In my memory, there was very little grass around the town. In fact, there was very little of anything green at all. Most things were grey because of the smoke that billowed from every chimney – both industrial and domestic – which was derived exclusively from coal. I remember, in particular, the walks back from Castleford's rugby league ground, on Wheldon Lane, in the early evenings of November when the dampness from the River Aire, the acrid exhaust fumes from the cars of the travelling away fans and the smoke from all the coal fires made a special type of smog, forever connected in my mind with rugby league.

When I was a young boy, already eager to be amongst fresh air and open spaces, there was one bit of green that gave me some hope. It was a patch of rough land behind our house. At the bottom of this patch of land was the railway line, which took trains from Castleford to Leeds. On one side it was bounded by the cemetery and on the other side by houses. It had been fenced off – after a fashion – and it lent itself to grazing for horses. There were not many horses in Castleford at that time, but the few that there were all seemed to find their way to this grazing and from a young toddler I became familiar with these gentle giants. At least they seemed giant to a little boy, and they were usually gentle.

The first horse I remember was a tough, black cob called Tommy. His job was to pull the roundabout, which you'd find in a part of the town where children's rides would appear from time to time. I can't remember the ride, but I do have some recollections of Tommy. One of my first full sentences as a tiny tot was, apparently, 'It horse hit me!'

I assume 'it horse' had knocked me over in his quest for extra carrots, or banged my bowl-haircut-head as he tossed his head in the air. I think I must have been a simple kid, or been very young, considering I used the word 'it' instead of 'the'. But my father ascribed this to my mishearing the Yorkshire habit of abbreviating 'the' to 't', as in 'I'm just going down t'pub to buy a ferret.'

I'm not convinced this was true, but it makes a nice story. And definitely 'it' horse made an impression on me because, according to my mother, I kept going on about it for months after, every time I saw Tommy. That same summer, 'it bee' also stung me and 'it other things' got me as well. The perils of toddlerhood.

After Tommy, a series of horses frequented the grass space behind our house, and I'm convinced that those early equine encounters contributed to my lifelong love of animals.

Some of these horses belonged to friends of my grandfather who were horsemen. John and Joe were brothers, huge and strong and impressive to a six-year-old me. They knew their horses inside out and loved them dearly. They would often bring horses to this patch of grassland over the summer. This made my dad happy because the grass was kept short and it looked tidier than an overgrown field. I was happy because I could play football, or even cricket, on flat, short grass rather than having to do battle with useless nettles and brambles. Mum was happy because she had the chance to feed apples and old bread to the horses, and fill up the old tin bathtub that doubled as a trough with buckets of water. Joe and John were happy because they had free grazing and knew that our family would keep half an eye on the well-being of their horses. Occasionally, one would escape through holes in the hedge or gaps in the wire fence. The marauding horse would variously end up in the middle of the roses, on the neighbour's lawn or even walking down the street, and I remember the great excitement that ensued as my dad gave chase.

As time went by, the brothers realised that while they had no proper experience, my mum and dad were good at looking after the horses and were therefore worthy custodians of their pregnant mares as they moved towards the end of their gestation period. The secluded field – assuming we could keep the horses contained and escapes infrequent – made a useful maternity unit. Every spring, a brood mare would arrive to sit out the final stages of her pregnancy under our care and in our field. To a budding young vet (although I didn't know that was my destiny at this point) awaiting the arrival of a newborn foal, gangly and precarious, was almost as exciting as waiting for Santa.

The first pregnant mare to take up temporary residence was Blossom. She was a lovely dapple-grey Shire horse, huge and imposing. Having learnt my lesson with Tommy, I was initially very careful around her, but we quickly became friends. I used to play cricket with my mates in the paddock in which she grazed. If I was lucky enough to connect with an over-pitched delivery (the ground was very uneven, on account of all the hoofprints, so the ball would turn sharply at random, making it hard to play shots off the front foot) Blossom was there, supervising at mid-on. She was calm and unfazed, even with flying cricket balls and shrieks from young children. She returned year on year, each time with a round, pregnant tummy. Annoyingly, Blossom always seemed to give birth during the night and without any warning, so I always missed the action. I'd run down to the field before school, with my carrots or bread to feed her, and I remember peering through the bushes, hoping to catch her in the act of giving birth. The closest I ever got was seeing a newly delivered foal, wobbling on its ridiculously long legs and looking for milk. Afterwards, my dad and I searched the field, looking for the afterbirth. I'd never seen anything like that before. It looked like a slimy sweatshirt, discarded as if used for a goalpost in one of our football games.

That was back in the seventies. I've seen thousands of afterbirths since those days in the field behind my house, and I've been lucky enough to be involved in countless births too. Missing out on seeing Blossom deliver her foals only served to whet my appetite. As with most things that happened over forty years ago, I've forgotten many of the details, but Blossom, her gentle disposition and the enigmatic arrival of her numerous foals on the rough cricket wicket lingers long in my memory.

By chance, I found myself in Kippax recently. I don't often venture back to West Yorkshire with work, but a donkey called Basil who had belonged to a client in Boroughbridge had just been sold to a smallholding in Kippax. The new arrival was intended as a companion for the various goats and pigs and a couple of horses. Basil needed to be castrated and, because I knew him, I offered to follow him to Kippax to do the honours. This was serendipitous because, when I was a kid in Castleford, Kippax was the furthest away place that I could see from my bedroom window. From the paddock where I set about getting Basil asleep and under anaesthetic, I could probably see my old bedroom if I looked hard enough. I could certainly see the railway line that ran along the northernmost edge of the field where I used to tend to Blossom.

Basil's operation went incredibly smoothly, which was a relief. Vets don't really like castrating donkeys. They don't respond quite so well as horses do to the drugs, and the procedure is a bit more complicated because there are bigger vessels running to each testicle. But Basil was fine and as we waited for him to recover from his anaesthetic, Tania, his new owner, brought out biscuits and cups of tea. It was a pleasant way to spend some time as the sun was shining and the various other animals on the farm came over to see what we were doing. The two goats and a pig came to join us as Tania and I leant on a gate and admired the view of my childhood home in the distance. I never like to leave a farm until the patient has woken up, so I had ample excuse to chat. I pointed out my parents' house to Tania, and recounted stories of Blossom and her foals.

'Well, that is an amazing coincidence,' said Tania, calmly but with obvious excitement, when I'd finished talking. 'You see that Shire horse over there? That dapple grey?' Tania paused momentarily before the final reveal: 'She is one of Blossom's foals! I've had her since she was a yearling. I got her from two brothers, one called Joe and the other called John. She's getting on now, of course. She must be over thirty years old.'

I looked at the magnificent Shire horse grazing contentedly in the nearby paddock. I wondered if I'd seen her before, but when she was just a few weeks old. She looked just like her mum.

Cheltenham and York

In my early days working in the Cotswolds, there were a lot of horses to look after. Most farms had a hunter or two in a stable in the yard alongside their sheep and cattle, and almost every house with a paddock had a horse of some description. Some were just for pleasure riding, while others were used for eventing, hunting or Pony Club. Then there were brood mares, whose athletic activities had been replaced by reproductive requirements, and racehorses, out of training or recovering from injury. Horses were everywhere and, during my time working there, there were several equine calls each day. This put me squarely outside my comfort zone, particularly because the retiring senior partner, whom I was supposed to be replacing, was highly regarded in the area as an equine expert. With his years of experience, booming voice and uber-long Volvo estate car, its boot bulging with bandages and bottles of 'bute', nobody ever questioned his diagnoses. He knew everyone and everyone knew him. He'd supervised pony camps and been one of the racecourse vets at the Cheltenham Festival for decades. A fresh-faced young cow vet from Yorkshire was always going to be up against it, but I tried my best.

'I want a second opinion,' was a phrase I quickly got used to when called upon to visit an expensive equine in a precarious position. At first, I genuinely presumed my inadequacies were real. I liked treating horses – in many ways they were like fast, good-looking cows, and were a lot less smelly and dirty. I some-times found their temperamental traits difficult to predict, however, probably because (apart from Tommy and Blossom and co.) I had not grown up around horses in the same way as some of my peers at vet school. I did not own a Puffa jacket and my wellies had steel toecaps and were grey and rugged, unlike the bottle green, calf-hugging variety favoured by, and obligatory for, any equine enthusiast. Despite this, I did have occasional successes, victorious battles in a long war of attrition.

One day, I was called to see an old horse suffering with colic. These cases are always stressful because, until you arrive, there is no way of knowing whether it is a mild bout of easy-to-treat spasmodic colic (where the long intestines go into painful spasm, often without obvious cause) or a catastrophic twist of the bowel, necessitating immediate euthanasia or very expensive and often risky surgery. There is a lot to decide in a short space of time and emotions always run high. In some ways, the decision-making process is actually quite straightforward. In practical terms, a horse with colic is either treated with drugs and laxatives by the attending vet, or it heads off to an equine hospital with capacity for surgical intervention or, if the prognosis is terrible and finances do not allow, euthanasia is performed.

At least, that's the theory and that's what I tell young vets when they head out to see their first equine colic case. In reality, of course, it is often much more complicated, and this was certainly the case when an elderly horse couldn't get up on the soft grassy slopes above Moreton-in-Marsh. Her owner was just as elderly and was quite rightly worried. The mare was rolling in griping pain, thrashing and kicking at her abdomen. My first job was to give her a sedative to numb some of the pain and start to stabilise the situation. Of course, an animal writhing in agony already presents a gloomy prospect, but on closer inspection things looked even worse. A heart rate of over eighty was more bad news. Heart rate rises with both pain and toxaemia. A normal horse has a heart rate of between thirty and forty beats per minute. The higher it is, the worse the outlook. Anything around a hundred is dire.

Next, I looked at the membranes in the mare's mouth. Severe colic causes damage to the bowel wall as the blood supply is compromised. This leads to the rapid development of toxaemia and the gums take on an unhealthy purple colouration, with what are called toxic rings above the teeth. There they were, pointing to one sad and inevitable outcome. I listened with my stethoscope to the intestinal sounds. Excessively loud noises indicate spasmodic colic – easily fixed. Reduced, or absent, sounds are bad, usually indicating an impaction or twist. As I expected, there was silence. I relayed all my findings to the owner as I went along. She said nothing, either ignoring my grave prognosis or not wanting to hear the gloomy news.

This completed the first stage of a basic colic examination. The next phase is more detailed, involving a rectal examination, the passing of a stomach tube if deemed necessary and a peritoneal tap, which is a method of sampling any fluid that might have developed in the abdomen. The presence of fluid is usually a bad thing. I carefully felt inside the recumbent horse's rectum. This procedure is not for the faint-hearted. A sudden movement or kick, in response to touching a tense and painful internal band of tissue, can have dire consequences for the vet's arm. Gingerly, I advanced my hand as far as it would go. Distended loops of bowel, like party balloons, stopped any further progress before I'd gone past the midpoint of my forearm. This all but confirmed a diagnosis of a twisted bowel. I retreated quickly to a safer place and explained all this to the owner, but she resolutely and stubbornly refused to believe me.

No surgeon would contemplate operating on such a severe case and I was certain there was no anaesthetist who would offer to help either. Again and again, I explained the grave situation to the headscarf-clad lady, but still she refused to believe there was no hope. Very politely, and I'm sure without any intention of undermining my professional advice, the old lady uttered the by now familiar phrase, 'I wonder if I could have another opinion?'

She went on, 'Maybe from those horse vets in Hook Norton? I know they are very good.'

I couldn't argue, although I was certain the outcome would be the same.

'Of course,' I said compliantly. 'I'll give them a ring.'

I injected yet another dose of painkiller to offer some sort of comfort to the stricken animal while we waited for the Hook Norton vet to arrive. The wait was about half an hour, which seemed just as uncomfortable for me as it was for the horse. I could have left and deferred all responsibility to the equine expert, but it didn't seem right to drive away at this moment of crisis. Eventually, a capable-looking four-wheel-drive vehicle appeared over the brow of the hill. I expected a huge, masculine horse vet with booming voice, checked shirt and trilby hat to step out. One who had the authority to pronounce a diagnosis and prognosis without even laying on a hand. Instead, the diminutive figure of a young female vet emerged. As she got closer, we recognised each other. Jane had been in the year below me at vet school and used to go out with my best mate. We hugged rather than shaking hands.

'Lovely to see you! How's it going? Are you busy? Is the new job good?' I asked, before turning to the matter in hand. Jane quickly confirmed the situation that I had described. Without raising an eyebrow, the elderly lady immediately agreed to Jane's plan, which was the same as mine. I drew up a large syringe of lethal injection. It was a sad end, but I couldn't help but smile slightly at the speed with which the words of the horse expert had been believed. Maybe she had the right wellies? Maybe it was the car?

One busy morning, an urgent visit to see a horse with choke demanded my attention. It fitted into a convenient round of calls, because the expensive eventer was at the stud adjacent to a large beef farm where I was scheduled to go and inspect a newly purchased bull. This, too, was an important job because the bull was a huge investment. His health and fertility needed to be assured and that was where I came in.

The choking horse was an emergency, so I rushed there first. It would be a short drive from Farlington Estate Stud on top of the hill down to see the new arrival at Farlington Manor Farm once I'd unclogged the horse's oesophagus. I pulled through the automatic, electric gates, which were flanked on either side by stone pillars, each topped with a huge stone horse's head. The sweeping drive with immaculate lawns and clipped trees on either side took me to the stable block. I'd been there just a few times before, for simple jobs like vaccinations and the occasional colic. A specialist stud vet visited on a regular basis to perform all the necessary fertility jobs, which were beyond the scope or remit of a normal mixed-practice vet and even beyond the scope of most standard horse vets. That said, my first ever visit to this impressive stud farm, in my first springtime working as a vet, had been a call to see a mare struggling to give birth; the stud had decided to bypass the specialist services of the stud vet in favour of our local practice as we were closer.

Being woken up in the middle of the night by the insistent bleep of a pager always increases the heart rate in an unhealthy fashion, but when I saw the message – *mare foaling* ASAP – my pulse rose another ten pips. The message was followed by the address at Farlington, which told me the patient was a horse worth several tens of thousands of pounds, and my heart rate went off the scale. That night, however, I was lucky. The exact details have been blurred by the fact that it was twenty-five years ago, and by the cortisol and adrenalin that surged through my veins as I drove to the yard, in the same way that the full details of giving birth to a baby are expunged from a mother's mind (although not so much from the mind of the anxious father, whose only function is holding a hand and the gas pipe). I was lucky because, by the time I arrived at Farlington Estate Stud in the small hours of that night in April, the mare was already licking her gangly baby, which in turn was already wobbling to its feet and looking for a teat.

Today's job would not find me so lucky. Choke is a distressing condition in which food, after being swallowed too quickly, forms an obstruction in the oesophagus. It's made worse if the food swells, for example if what is eaten is unsoaked sugar beet. The horse panics – and so does the owner, because green and brown, gloopy and slimy liquid issues unnaturally from the mouth and nostrils. A horse with a bad case of choke looks like the end of the world, and it can be exactly that for the horse if correct treatment is not put in place.

I was shown into the plush American-style barn, where each

stable's oak door had the occupant's name etched perfectly in the centre. Apart from the pool of turbid discharge in front of the suffering young mare, there was not a trace of dirt or detritus anywhere and the stud oozed wealth.

'She was absolutely fine yesterday!' the groom bellowed, anxious and stressed. She was obviously very worried and I sensed that the sight of me arriving, rather than the usual horse expert, had raised her concern to another level. I was getting used to this by now!

I started asking various questions, trying to work out a possible cause.

'We found her this morning. I went to bring her in from the paddock for the farrier who's coming later. I can't understand it. There's absolutely NO chance she's eaten anything other than grass and her hay net!' She was adamant.

But a diet of grass alone should not cause choke, so there was an unsolved mystery. I sedated the mare and set about feeding a large, plastic tube up her nose. In horses, this is the way to pass a stomach tube, or any tube for that matter. An endoscope goes up the nose too and then down into the lungs, looking for signs of infection or airway disease. A stomach tube goes the same way, but needs to be swallowed as it arrives at the throat, so it can progress down the oesophagus towards the stomach. It can form part of the examination of a horse with colic and can also allow liquids to be administered – lubricants or laxatives, for example – if the problem is an impaction.

My aim today was to reach the obstruction – whatever it was – with my pipe, then introduce volumes of warm water. A combination of dissolution and physical flushing usually clears the problem. It's a complicated process for several reasons. A stressed horse, even under sedation, resents both the intubation and the fluid being instilled. Head-tossing, foot-stomping and nose-snorting is common. The process takes at least half an hour and sometimes has to be repeated several times, so it is no quick fix. An additional problem is that the delicate nasal structures have a large blood supply that, if disturbed, can bleed profusely. The addition of blood makes the torrid scene even more grotesque and, although not usually serious, only adds to everyone's anxiety.

After several buckets of water, I had made little progress. The mare was upset and the groom was too.

'Are you sure this is right?' she shouted, obviously worried about the horse under her care and my lack of progress. 'Why aren't you making her better? Could it be something else? We've never had anything like this before.' Expecting another demand for a second opinion, I pre-empted this by offering another plan.

'I'm going to give her a relaxant injection to ease any spasm in the oesophagus, and then I'll come back in about an hour and have another go,' I explained. Often choke cases needed a second and sometimes third visit. I could drop down the hill, see my bull and come back for round two with my tube. This plan seemed to meet with approval and I washed the nasal blood from my hands and arms and headed down the lane that connected Farlington Stud to Farlington Manor Farm. It was a public road, but since it was entirely contained within the parkland of the estate, I'd never seen any traffic on it, other than tractors, quad bikes or horses, and it was a scenic drive.

'Sorry I'm late,' I said when I arrived to see the bull, and explained what had held me up.

'Those horses are a damned nuisance,' exclaimed the farmer. 'They insist on putting them on the same grazing as our cattle. The greedy ones stick their heads in the feed troughs and eat all our cattle food. It's not as if they need any free charity food from us! I keep telling them to keep them out, but you know horse owners – always think they know best!'

I smiled and dealt with the new arrival, who was handsome and grand, taking measurements along with samples of blood and faeces to test for disease. I was done quickly and headed back to have another attempt at treating the horse, who looked a little better, despite having a stain of blood on her nostril.

'I'll put a tube in again and see if we can flush it out completely this time,' I said. 'Is there any chance this mare could have had access to any cattle food?'

The groom apologetically raised a hand to her mouth.

'Yes, there is!' came the reply as the reality dawned. 'We graze them in the same field as some cattle. They could have eaten some calf feed.'

I applied more water and eventually it ran in freely and the blockage was gone. Horse vet or not, I was relieved to have solved the mystery and fixed the mare!

Evening surgery had just finished and I was the lucky vet going home with the beeper in his pocket. It was soon in action, alerting me to a lame horse. It sounded serious, as any out-of-hours visit to see a lame animal usually is. When I arrived, the owner was waiting in his drive. He had a bald head and a ruddy, hypertensive complexion. The sharp suit and shiny shoes told me he must have spent his day in the centre of Leeds, maybe completing important business deals or prosecuting at the Crown Court. My arrival did not seem to lower his blood pressure, or ease the redness of his face. Even before I'd had chance to examine the patient, I sensed another (yes, *another*) second opinion would be required.

I was shown to a paddock behind the house. It was more of a hall than a house. The expansive grounds swept away from a beautiful orangery down towards the Wolds. The views were magnificent, especially as the sun was just starting to set over

the dales towards the western horizon. While the view was spectacular and the impending sunset calming, none of it rubbed
off on me. The expensive-looking, slender thoroughbred stood
miserably on the slope beside the croquet lawn, its left forelimb
hanging limp and useless. Even from a distance, I knew it was
serious and that the leg was certainly broken. There's not much
else that makes a horse sweat while standing on three legs. If I
was right, there would be a serious discussion to be had, with
only one logical conclusion. It would be the end of a dream for
the novice racehorse owner.

The poor horse was obviously in a lot of pain and, on closer
examination, I could see the left front leg waving ineffectually
in the breeze. The filly had obviously slipped on the bank and
fractured her humerus (the bone between the elbow and
shoulder). Frustratingly for me, as a young and fresh-faced vet,
these bone breaks are very difficult to demonstrate to the owner.
The strong muscles around the upper part of the limb go into
spasms of contraction in an attempt to stabilise the fracture and
minimise the pain. It is the body's natural reaction and it helps
the patient, but it makes the job harder for the vet, especially
without the aid of a portable, digital X-ray machine (which had
not yet been invented). It also makes it infinitely more challenging to persuade the businessman, non-horseman owner that
there is anything more serious than a muscle strain. A break near
the bottom of the limb is often unequivocal – the normal anatom-
ical rigidity is replaced by an unnatural floppiness that is
impossible to not spot as it freakishly defies the pillars of
normality; but higher up the limb, it is not so obvious.

This evening's owner could not be convinced that there was
any deviance from normal anatomy, and flatly refused to believe
my diagnosis of a fracture around the yearling's elbow.

I tried my best to recommend immediate euthanasia but,

though my efforts to demonstrate the seriousness of the problem and its cause were unimpeachable, the businessman uttered words I'd heard before, insisting: 'I'd like a second opinion!'

The sun disappeared behind the hills as I dialled the number of a nearby specialist equine practice to explain the situation. They assured me that their on-call vet would be on his way shortly. I hoped I was correct as I administered a large dose of painkiller, before answering another call. There would be no peace for me this evening, so I made my excuses and left the filly to the expert.

The following morning, I phoned the owner to check the result of the second opinion. I left a message on his phone. He was either busy or avoiding my call. Next, I called the equine practice. Luckily, the same vet was still around after his night on call and came to the phone. I smiled to myself, knowing that he, too, had probably been up all night – or at least had a fitful night's sleep awaiting colic calls and second opinions for owners who didn't believe their own vet.

'Oh yes,' he said wearily. 'A fractured distal humerus. A classic. No need for X-rays, it was a simple diagnosis.'

I was relieved I'd got it right, but frustrated – not the first or last time – that I had not been believed. The equine vet continued, without any provocation or suggestion from me, 'And that owner! What a tosser!'

Blessed is the veterinary surgeon who manages to maintain a successful career working with horses. It's not easy!

Donkey Sagas

I had been treating some of the animals at Cannon Hall Farm for a few months. The farm was somewhat out of the practice's usual catchment area, but since it was just a stone's throw from the major trunk road that is the M1 and the practice at Boroughbridge was situated close to the A1, it only actually took about fifty minutes from door to door. This was not much longer than it might take to get to some of the outlying farms at the top of Nidderdale, on the edge of the Wolds or nestling in the foothills of the North York Moors, so visits to attend some of the challenging cases at Cannon Hall were eminently feasible for me.

I got to know the Nicholson family, who farmed at Cannon Hall Farm, through my involvement with the Channel 5 series *Springtime on the Farm*, which was filmed there, and in which I featured as a sort of 'presenter'. I put the term in inverted commas because I am really a vet and not really a presenter. Nevertheless, I got to sit in the green room and talk with proper TV people.

While we were filming some VTs for *Springtime* (pre-recorded pieces of footage, to be inserted into the 'live' show), I was shown Gary the donkey. To be more accurate, what I was actually shown was Gary the donkey's penis.

'What do you think of this?' asked Robert, one of the farming brothers, who was anxious about his stud. Gary was a tall, strong and proud entire male donkey, used to getting his own way and to getting his oats. I bent over and tried to peer at the penis from a distance. Donkeys are notoriously good at kicking, and I wanted to get a good look before doing anything else. I could make out a plum-sized mass on the side of his prepuce – the folded skin around his penis. Its surface was ulcerated and it had apparently grown rapidly. These were hallmarks of a cancerous growth. Robert's brother, David, was tending to the other donkeys (all either members of Gary's harem or immediate family) in a nearby pen, and came over to help.

'I'd like to have a feel. Can you hold him? Is he likely to kick?' I asked, hoping that he would be calm but expecting he might be the opposite.

'Julian, I think there's quite a good chance he will,' advised Robert. 'It's tender and he's a headstrong kind of donkey.'

'You'd better make sure you've got nice warm hands, Julian,' quipped David, ever the joker. It wasn't a bad idea.

Once Gary had been caught and restrained, and after I had rubbed my hands together for several minutes to warm them up, as David had suggested, I carefully reached under the donkey's tummy and edged my fingers along until I felt the sheath. Gary looked very relaxed, but I held my breath, ready to leap out of the way should he change his mind. The mass was not good, though. Hard and ulcerated, it had all the features of malignancy that I had suspected when I saw it from a distance. It was probably a squamous cell carcinoma or maybe a sarcoid. Either way, it was bad. However, the lump was dangling on a thin stalk, about as wide as my little finger. This gave me some hope.

'It doesn't feel very good, lads,' I explained. 'It's likely to be a cancerous growth and it will need to be removed.'

Robert and David looked concerned. I knew that look. It was the look that appeared on the face of any Yorkshire farmer when the idea of surgical intervention was broached. I could see worry in the depths of their eyes, as if enormous pound signs pervaded their peripheral vision.

'But it's okay, because I have a plan,' I added, to put them out of their pecuniary misery.

'This lump is on a stalk and I think I can fix it by applying some rubber rings around its base. You know, like the rubber rings used to castrate lambs?'

I hoped this solution would be simple and painless, free of risk and free of huge expense. I would need to sedate Gary, instil some local anaesthetic into the skin around the base of the mass and then apply the stretched ring around it, so it tightened around the stalk. The blood supply would shrivel up over the coming weeks and then, in theory, the lump should fall off.

'That sounds like a grand plan,' said Robert, content that I'd offered a sensible solution. I arranged to get everything I would need and then a date was booked to place the rings on Gary's penis.

On the day of the 'op', Gary was as frisky as ever. He was the biggest donkey I'd ever seen. He had long, strong legs and a solid frame and he towered above the female donkeys in the barn where they all lived. With his obstinate characteristics, he had similarities to a camel! As I gathered my equipment, I hoped I would be able to make a more thorough assessment of the problem area. David had a plan to encourage Gary's huge penis to expose itself to its full extent, and thereby facilitate a more detailed examination and make treatment easier.

'My plan, Julian,' he explained, 'is to bring Jenny into this pen. She's a very attractive female donkey and I think she'll be just the job to persuade Gary to extend his willy, if you know what I mean. That way you should be able to give him a proper examination.' It sounded like a fair plan.

Moments later, Jenny was led into the large pen. We stood back and waited. It didn't take long to achieve the effect we needed. Oblivious to the problem on his penis, Gary very quickly and furiously attempted to mate with Jenny. This was good for me, because I could inspect the length of his penis easily, but it was not so good for Jenny. She was neither in season nor in the mood, and kicked poor Gary in the chest with both her back feet, in the classic 'kicking like a mule' way that you might see in a children's cartoon. Luckily, the donkey's pride was only slightly dented and there was no physical injury. He had thick skin and tough muscles on his chest – and I guessed he was quite accustomed to rejection of this kind. We corralled him into a corner to catch him with a headcollar. I hoped he would cooperate with my efforts.

After a moment or two of struggling, I managed to administer a sedative injection and Gary started to look drowsy. The next job was to inject a syringe of local anaesthetic into the base of the lump. This was the bit I was looking forward to least. Local anaesthetic, as anyone accident-prone will know, stings like mad when it is first injected, a bit like a bad insect bite. It only lasts for a moment, but I expected that, even under sedation, Gary would let rip with a hind foot, aiming at the imagined biting fly, which was actually my head. And this is exactly what he did. Luckily, it was a much more half-hearted attempt to cause serious injury than Jenny's double-barrel kick had been earlier and my progress was not disturbed. The first bit of local is the worst and, once that area of skin is rendered numb, more can be instilled without much more discomfort. I was soon ready to go with my rings.

The little orange rings, like tiny rubber doughnuts, fit onto a special metal applicator, which has four prongs. When the handles are squeezed, the four prongs expand outwards and this makes the aperture in the middle of the donut expand to a size big enough to fit over a fifty-pence piece. This was also big enough to fit over the penile growth. I stretched a ring over the tumour, pushing it as high up as I could to ensure I'd got it all. It worked perfectly and I placed another couple for good measure. Then all we needed to do was wait. Once the blood supply had been occluded, it should shrivel up and fall off. The lump, I mean. Not the penis.

'That, Julian, is a brilliant job!' exclaimed Robert, delighted that we had solved the problem without incurring too much risk or expense. 'I love a simple solution and that is straight out of a Herriot book!'

I patted Gary on his huge nose and headed back to my car, hopeful that my rubber rings would solve the problem. I promised to keep in touch with the brothers at Cannon Hall about Gary's progress.

A few weeks later, everything looked good. The tumour had dropped off and the small, sore patch that was all that remained was healing nicely. Gary was back in action, furiously working to expand his herd. Once I had checked the patient, Robert ushered me into a large, adjacent pen.

'Julian, come and meet Julian,' he called over his shoulder. 'He's Gary's latest offspring, born yesterday!' They had named one of his babies after me! I was touched – until it became clear that a name change was needed. The fluffy baby with its enormous ears was a girl. David, in his excitement, had forgotten to check. And so Julian hastily became Julia – but it was still a kind thought!

Eventually, normal donkey life at Cannon Hall was re-established, and the future for Gary seemed rosy. However, some months later, I received a worried message from Robert. The growth, which we had all thought was gone for good, had now reappeared.

This was ominous news because it suggested the mass was more aggressive than I'd previously thought. There must have been tendrils of tumour cells running up through the stalk. It also meant that more invasive surgery would be needed. Anaesthetics, scalpels, expense and risk were now on the table, although I knew full well that the brothers' devotion to Gary, as with all their animals, would overcome any cost issues.

I talked through what I'd need to do next. We would have to use Gary's barn as a makeshift operating theatre, and I would have to bring in some help to supervise the anaesthetic. I made a call to Matt, who was Cannon Hall's local vet. I'd met him before. He is another of those people who have boundless energy and enthusiasm and we had immediately hit it off. I was delighted when he agreed to help me with Gary.

D-day (donkey day) arrived and Matt and I arrived at the same time, to plan and prepare for the surgery. As ever, I had a camera crew following my every move. I checked with Matt that he didn't mind as not everyone likes to have their work scrutinised on national television, but it was a great story and I felt sure that the tense surgery on Gary's private parts would be exactly what the series producer and the post-production team of *The Yorkshire Vet* wanted. Fortunately, Matt relished the opportunity both to help the donkey and to show off his veterinary prowess on camera.

Everyone got ready. Matt was in charge of the injections and making sure Gary was properly asleep. I was the surgeon and concentrated hard on making accurate incisions and removing every trace of tumour. There was a lot that could go wrong and I couldn't disguise the tremor in my hand as I prepared for the first cut. I'm not usually nervous when I'm working, but today I felt much more pressure than usual.

But I need not have feared, because things went extremely smoothly – everything was straight out of the textbook, in fact. The anaesthetic was perfect and the surgery was slick. The tumour was off – hopefully completely this time – and Gary was back on his feet in no time. Matt had acquitted himself with aplomb, both in his professional capacity and in front of the camera.

I quickly recognised in him all the qualities a young vet should have. He was passionate about his job; relaxed, light-hearted and even comical when appropriate, but caring throughout. He was youthful, smiley and handsome. Most importantly for viewers of *The Yorkshire Vet*, he had a sufficient Yorkshire twang to be a veterinary TV star of the future. I hoped I wouldn't need to see Gary again, at least not in relation to his mass. Matt, on the other hand, I felt sure I would see much more of in the future . . .

I had donkeys on my mind that summer, even after Gary had been sorted out. Mabel and Doris were donkeys in need of a new home. Their elderly owners were no longer able to look after them and had contacted a donkey rescue charity for help. The charity had requested that the donkeys underwent some blood tests to check for underlying health issues before proceeding, and that's where I came in. I duly took the samples as instructed, but as I packaged up the tubes of blood, ready to post them to the lab, I couldn't help thinking that I could do more. I wondered if *I* might be able to find the pair of donkeys a new home.

Steve and Jeanie Green were old friends. I visited their traditional old farm almost every week throughout my first twenty years in practice. They had cows and cats in abundance and also a donkey called Horace, who was part of the fixtures and fittings at Stoneybrough Farm. His greying nose was often visible over the rickety wooden stable door when I visited to see a cow down with milk fever, or a calf with respiratory disease. I'd known Horace for most of my veterinary career. From the safety of his stable, or from a nearby pasture, he'd cast an eye over much of my clinical work at Jeanie's farm, occasionally vocalising his disapproval, bellowing the classic 'Hew Haw' for which donkeys are famous.

But Horace, like everything and everyone, eventually succumbed to old age. Old age and, apparently, an overdose of carrots fed to him by a well-meaning neighbour over the fence. Horace's demise had left a donkey-sized hole at Stoneybrough. So, when I met Mabel and Doris and realised their circumstances, I couldn't help thinking that they would make a great addition to the Greens' family. I broached the idea to their owners first. They were more than happy with the prospect of the pair finding a new home nearby. I called Jean, who was delighted that she might have a replacement for Horace. I felt like Cupid on a Valentine's mission to ignite a long-term and loving relationship. But (to mix metaphors) like Cinderella before the ball, none of this would happen if I couldn't manage to arrange some transport.

As chance would have it, this was more straightforward than I'd expected. The day after my matchmaking, I happened to be lambing a ewe on a farm I hadn't been to before. Everyone there was excited to meet me, because they'd seen me on telly! As I untangled the mal-presented lamb, conversation quickly turned to television matters.

'We really love it when the Greens are on!' exclaimed Ian as he held onto the sheep's head while I worked away. 'What an interesting farming family they are, we'd love to meet them!'

Just at that moment, I spotted a pony trailer on the far side of the farmyard and another plan came into my head.

By the time I'd delivered the lamb, it was all arranged. Ian and his daughters would collect the donkeys from the elderly couple and deliver them to Steve and Jeanie. They'd get to meet their TV heroes and I had my donkey transport. Everything had fallen into place.

Mabel and Doris arrived at Stoneybrough the following week, just in time for a big occasion. It was a special wedding anniversary for Steve and Jeanie. A pair of donkeys was an unusual gift!

'It's good to have some donkeys back on the farm,' said Jeanie with a smile as Mabel and Doris tottered down the ramp of the trailer and into their new paddock. 'You can't beat a good old donkey!'

I was happy in the certain knowledge that Mabel and Doris were in loving and capable hands.

Foalings

I remember watching an episode of *All Creatures Great and Small* one Sunday evening when I was eight or nine years old. Tristan had recently started work with Siegfried Farnon and James Herriot and, fresh out of vet school, was full of enthusiasm for the challenges of veterinary life. The huge, old telephone rang in Skeldale House, the veterinary surgery where the stories were based. It was a worried farmer. He was, quite rightly, anxious about his mare, who was struggling to deliver a foal. In those days, a horse was as integral a part of a mixed farm as a Border Collie and, even when I started my veterinary career several decades later, the sight of a horse peering over a creaking stable door in the farmyard was a common one.

On the programme, a discussion ensued between Herriot, Siegfried Farnon and newbie Tristan, who leapt up in a rush, intent on solving the problem with the horse.

'But it has a head back, Tristan. It's not an easy case for your first foaling,' warned Herriot. 'It's a tough job – are you up to it or shall I go?'

Needless to say, Tristan jumped at the challenge, even though it was sure to be very difficult. I remember watching this scene and marvelling that there was such a career – a way of life in which you would be faced with life-and-death challenges like this on a daily basis. And all in the fresh magical beauty of the Yorkshire countryside! To get to call it work must surely be invigorating.

Approximately fifteen years later, having graduated from vet school and with a head full of theory, I found myself in a similar position to Tristan as I faced the prospect of my first foaling. It was about one o'clock in the morning in the early part of May and I was rudely awakened by my beeper. A farmer had a mare struggling to give birth. Unlike Tristan, I had no senior colleague offering to go in my place. Not that I wanted that anyway. I was following in the veterinary footsteps of my childhood hero and I had been waiting for this moment since I had been offered a place at vet school!

I knew where to go, although I had only been to the farm on a handful of occasions. Once I'd gone to see a cow with mastitis and another time one with a condition called 'silage eye'. I had also lambed a couple of ewes there. My cattle and sheep jobs had gone well and I felt I was well on my way up the steep climb towards achieving the reputation of being a decent vet. Tonight's job would be a much bigger challenge than my previous visits, though, and there was a lot at stake – the life of the mare, the life of the as yet unborn foal and the trust of the farming family. I crossed my fingers.

I was nervous. As a veterinary student, it is easy to become adept at lambing sheep or calving cows. Sheep farmers are always happy to get the help of a young student at lambing time. There is a lot of work to be done, and a farm with several hundred sheep is a perfect place to learn one end of a lambing rope from another. Out of a flock of five hundred sheep, somewhere between fifty and a hundred might need assistance in some form. It's a similar case with cows, although because it is unusual to have several hundred cows giving birth in a short period of time, experience is harder to acquire. I was lucky to have spent a full month as a student working on a busy dairy farm in Dorset, where I had helped with dozens of calvings.

But horses are altogether a different kettle of fish (so to speak). Firstly, unless you happen to be based at a busy stud in Newmarket, horses tend to be kept in smaller numbers. They never have twins (or, at least, it is very, very rare), so there is no chance that assistance will be required to untangle the legs of two babies trying to exit the birth canal at the same time, as often happens in sheep. The other issue making it difficult to acquire the skills of delivering a foal is that, just like the process of conception in the horse, it is very rapid, if not to say explosive. Without problems, foals are delivered in a matter of a few minutes, rather than the protracted affair common in other species. All these things make it difficult to get experience foaling mares, as a student or even as a qualified veterinary surgeon. And, to make matters harder and more stressful for the vet, when things go wrong, they usually go very badly wrong.

Some months after that first foaling, I heard on the grapevine about some advice a vet acquaintance of mine was once given by a seasoned colleague on this subject.

'The first thing I always do when I get called to foal a mare,' the seasoned individual explained, 'is to have a cup of tea.'

My acquaintance was somewhat shocked and surprised at this story, as was I. True, some 'emergency' visits are not real emergencies. A dog with diarrhoea that has splattered the kitchen during the night, or a sheep with a smelly discharge, for example, need sorting promptly, but they do not compare to the absolute, immediate urgency of an impending foaling.

'Well, under normal circumstances it all happens so quickly,' the experienced vet had gone on. 'If you dawdle for five minutes or more, the foal has usually come out by itself. It really does save you a job.'

It was hard to imagine subscribing to this maverick approach, and so I never have. Just like Tristan, I always drop everything to attend to a horse giving birth.

And this evening I felt just like him as I rushed along the silent rural roads of North Yorkshire. Even though it was early summer and the nights were getting shorter, it was very dark. Mares always seem to have their babies at the quietest time and in the most secluded place. They are sensitive and secretive souls and don't like to have people watching.

I arrived at the farm and pulled my car alongside the barn door, from where a light was shining. This was surely where the action would be. I went in to investigate. There was a central fold yard, full of about a dozen dozing cows. Some were sitting comfortably and ruminating. A couple were standing by the ring feeder, munching on silage. They were all pregnant too, patiently waiting to give birth before joining the rest of the herd outside to enjoy the grass. These were the 'stragglers' – the last few cows left at the end of the spring calving, who had calved late the previous year and had therefore become pregnant after their herd-mates.

The fold yard should really have been empty by now, sheep lambed and cows calved and all outside thriving in the fields, so that the farmer could concentrate on the serious issue of her three pregnant brood mares.

And that was exactly what Diane was doing. She was giving the mare her full attention. She had arranged a twenty-four-hour surveillance system for her favourite horse and was in position in a deckchair covered in blankets, opposite the stable door. A flask of coffee and a part-empty bottle of whisky sat within reach of her right hand, suggesting that this was where she had been reclining for many hours, while a metal bucket full of warm water steamed on the other side of the chair, with a towel folded neatly over the chair arm. Nowadays, technology has taken over and farmers and horse owners often have CCTV systems installed so they can supervise from the comfort of the kitchen, or even the pub, by means of an app on their phone. But in the mid-nineties, farmers either got up every hour or so, or napped with their stock. Diane fell into the latter camp, preferring to stay with her charge. Looking at the part-empty bottle of whisky, I suspected the option of waking up every hour, getting dressed and leaving the warmth of the farmhouse was not a system that would work for her.

'Ah, it's you, Julian. I hope you're feeling fit,' she said by way of a greeting as she clambered out of her deckchair and adjusted her woolly hat. The middle of the night can still be a cold time in May.

'Morning. What's the problem?' I asked, wondering if it was a pointless question.

'Well, she's been waxed up for about a week – that's when I started sleeping in this chair – but it all started about an hour ago. She's agitated and she's up and down and trying to push, but I'm worried she's not making any progress,' Diane explained.

'Waxing up' is not a special depilation technique for horses, but a term that describes changes that occur in the udder when a mare is close to the point of giving birth. The gestation period can be very unpredictable and so it can be difficult to know the exact due date. I peered over the stable door. The mare was lying down, puffing, pushing and then standing up again, clearly agitated. Equally clear was that I needed to get to work.

Diane went into the stable. She was an expert with her horses and the brood mare was visibly calmed by her soothing words as she took hold of the headcollar. By now the mare was standing up, but I couldn't see anything protruding from her vulva. I couldn't delay my internal examination any further. I was anxious, not only about what I might find or how I might solve the problem, but about whether the horse might kick or twist vigorously at the wrong moment. As gently as I could, with plenty of lubricant on my hand and arm, I made my first tentative exploration.

It didn't go well. The mare immediately flung herself to the ground as another wave of contractions started. Her legs thrashed and waved dangerously. A horse in pain, writhing and rolling on the floor, is not very safe, especially in the confines of a stable. Cows can be corralled into a cattle crush or restrained behind a gate, and on stud units horses are placed in 'stocks' to provide a safer place to perform an examination, but I had no such luxury tonight.

I knelt down to have a second go. My hand slid in easily at first, but vigorous straining resumed as soon as I was in past my elbow and I started to worry that there was a real chance of sustaining a broken arm. There was one obvious foot but nothing else, and my heart sank. In cattle, from where I was drawing my experience, the head follows closely behind the front feet. Foals have much longer legs, so the head is further in. This dawned on me at that very moment and I eased further in. Between lurches and contractions, I managed to ascertain the problem. I could feel a nose. This was good news and meant the challenge would hopefully be less than Tristan's had been, forty-five years earlier. The other good news was that I could feel the second front leg. It was flexed at the carpus (in horsey terminology, bent at the knee), and this was what was causing the obstruction.

I knew what I needed to do next, which was to flip the lower part of the leg forward, straightening it out so both front legs were together. It sounds simple, but it wasn't. The lower part of the leg was long and the space in the mare's pelvis was limited. Against all the strength of the mare's uterine contractions, I had to push the errant leg further in to give me some more space and then hook the foot up, all the time avoiding her kicks and attempts to stand up. I huffed and puffed and tried not to swear, and eventually everything was lined up.

The next job was to pull. The mare was tired and I wanted to get the foal out as soon as I could, so I attached ropes to each leg and connected my calving sticks. These are short pieces of broom handle that make it easier to apply pressure to the ropes. I took both to start with and assumed my place lying behind the mare, pulling as if I was trying to unearth a giant root vegetable. It was hard and I pulled and pulled, while all the time Diane whispered and soothed her horse at the head end, like a husband in a maternity ward. Eventually the foal was out, leggy and slimy and alive! I'd done it! I'd delivered my first ever foal!

'Well done, Julian!' Diane beamed, letting the new mother get on with her maternal duties, licking the foal, as she rushed to give me a hug.

'I think we deserve a drink!' she said, pulling the cork out of her whisky bottle. We had done well and I was delighted. It was nothing compared to Tristan's first foaling, but I had a warm feeling inside me, which was only in small part thanks to the whisky.

Some years later, Diane told me about another animal she had been supervising as it waited to give birth. She related the story over a cup of coffee one day after I had been to vaccinate her horses and pregnancy test a few of her cows.

'Julian, it was very funny,' she said, chuckling, as her face got redder and redder. 'I'd got up to check a cow that was calving. We'd been waiting for her for days and I'd got fed up with checking her every couple of hours through the night, so I came out at first light. I thought I'd only be up for a few minutes so I didn't bother to get dressed – I just put on my wellies.'

I already had a disturbing image of a naked farmer's wife wearing only a pair of muddy wellies as she blithely opened the front door and made the twenty- or thirty-yard walk to the farm buildings.

'The cow was fine and so I turned round and came back inside. At the very moment I got to the front door, for some reason I looked up at the electricity pylon that was on the edge of that paddock over there' – she pointed out of one of the kitchen windows – 'and there was a MAN on the pylon, doing some checks, and he'd seen me walking around my farm stark-bollock naked!' By now Diane was barely able to speak for laughter and so was I.

'The next day there were about five men!' she added.

There is another equine veterinary emergency associated with foaling. A retained placenta occurs when the membranes that provided nourishment to the developing foal fail to detach after the foal has been delivered. Just as is the case in humans, in horses if the placenta is not passed quickly, all sorts of serious problems can develop.

For a horse vet, a call at first light between March and May often means a placenta has been retained and, while it is probably acceptable to have a cup of tea before leaving the house, it is sufficiently urgent to mean no breakfast.

The first retained placenta I ever treated, soon after I had started practising, was that very six o'clock in the morning, pre-breakfast call. The farm was just like Diane's, with the old, brick-lined fold yard with low arches typical of most traditional Yorkshire farms, and more conducive to housing cattle than horses. There were several ponies in the yard, happily and comfortably munching on hay. My patient, however, had her mind on matters more important than hay, because her new baby was already on its feet, getting acquainted with its gangly legs and looking for milk. The afterbirth hung ominously from the mare's vulva. It should have detached almost immediately after the foal had landed. Its persistence was a big problem, because it offered a route for ascending infection. Sepsis and toxaemia could follow, resulting in all sorts of complications, one of which was death. The seriousness of a retained placenta in a horse was drilled into us as veterinary students. It was serious on a whole different level than the same condition in a cow or sheep.

The course of action was also drilled into us – gentle, manual removal using the fingers to carefully tease apart the membrane from its attachment inside the uterus. I can still remember my obstetrics lecturer, Dr Jackson, with his arm outstretched, his fingers gently wiggling and his eyes closed in concentration as he demonstrated what to do. Sometimes uterine irrigation was required to flush the membranes out. In cases where there was concern about the completeness of the removal, or if the attachment was too firm, the next course of action was to give a dose of the hormone oxytocin to release milk from the udder and make the uterus contract back down to its small, pre-pregnancy size. A suckling neonate stimulates production of the mother's natural oxytocin, but in cases like this, extra help is required.

So, just like Dr Jackson had instructed that day in the lecture theatre in his smart shoes and clean white lab coat, I carefully inserted my hand and wiggled my gloved and lubricated fingers to separate the layers. It seemed to be working and after about ten tense minutes, the sticky placental membranes were on the straw floor. I stretched the membranous structure out so I could inspect it for completeness. I once did this with the placenta of an alpaca. It looked like a pair of pink running leggings and it made me chuckle. It's funny when things in a veterinary medicine context look like something completely different – but, amusing as it might be to inspect a placenta, it's actually very important to ensure it is all present and correct. If even a trace is left inside, that can be just as dangerous. I couldn't be certain I'd got it all out, so the mare would need some oxytocin. I knew this powerful drug needed to be used with great care in the horse. The dose was tiny but even so, if injected by the intravenous route, it would have to be given very slowly. That was the other thing that I remembered from that obstetrics lecture in the dusty old surroundings of Cambridge Vet School. The bold capital letters in my obstetrics notes urged caution. With Dr Jackson's firm but gentle warnings still ringing in my ears, I drew up the correct dose and aimed for the pony's jugular. The flashback of dark blood was immediate – this was good. I'd hit the vein first time. Slowly, slowly I trickled the small volume of colourless liquid into the pony, pausing every few seconds to draw back on the syringe, checking and rechecking that my needle was still in the vein.

What happened next took me by surprise. After just a few moments, the pony suddenly flung herself in the air, did a backflip and landed in a heap in the (thankfully) deep straw bedding, narrowly missing her foal. The poor mare shook and convulsed on the floor and I thought I had killed her. The foal looked on, surprised. The owner stared in horror.

'What the heck is happening?' she screamed, convinced that her mare, who moments earlier had been standing comfortably with her baby suckling contentedly, was now about to die.

Of course, I was panicking internally. What on earth had I done? Was the pony actually about to die? If so, it would be a terrible start to my day and a horrible end to the pony's life. I tried to stay calm and attempted to offer some reassurance.

'Yes, this is, of course, a completely normal reaction to the drug,' I bluffed, trying not to let my voice shake. 'The mare will be fine. It's just the uterus contracting. Don't worry!'

I quickly grabbed another bottle, this one containing very strong painkiller, and fumbled for a syringe. It was obviously a lame attempt at explaining the problem, so I tried to add a bit more detail: 'It's a bit like period pains.' At this point I realised I had overstepped the mark and had entered an area about which I genuinely knew nothing. I decided to shut up, and drew up the dose of painkiller.

Within a few moments, which felt like hours, everything was back to normal. I'd managed to inject the painkiller and the mare was soon standing, calm and relaxed. The foal was happily suckling again, rather than watching its mother in the throes of death, and the final fragments of murky pink placenta were all out and safely buried in the muck heap.

I waved goodbye to the now relieved owner and the healthy patients. There didn't seem to be any ill feeling and it had, apart from one minor and temporarily very stressful hiatus, been a successful procedure. I sat in the car and took a few breaths to gather myself after the trauma. I checked my pulse, which was slowing back to approximately normal. I also checked the time. It was ten to eight. There was time to go home for breakfast before starting the rest of my working day.

At home, I put on the kettle and put bread in the toaster, then made a beeline for my obstetrics notes. My eyes skimmed past the bovine and ovine sections, each with their own warnings and provisos and capital letters, before I found *EQUINE OBSTETRICS*. I flicked through the pages, fingering each line, until I found the section on the dose and administration of oxytocin for a horse.

Oxytocin, read the heading. The dose *was* correct. According to the notes, I had done everything right . . . but, in large letters, just below the dose details, it said: *Often causes colic signs. ALWAYS WARN THE OWNER!*

Once again, Dr Jackson had been right, and I'd learnt another lesson. This one in practice rather than in a stuffy lecture theatre.

5. Cats

Animal owners often say you are either a 'dog person' or a 'cat person'. Until the summer of 1988, all of my family fell firmly into the dog category. The closest any of us Nortons came to cuddling cats was when I volunteered to foster a litter of newborn kittens, rescued from dire straits by the RSPCA. I had been working with a whirling dervish of energy called Gail, who was a veterinary nurse and also helped with the animal charity. Gail had taken me under her wing for a couple of weeks during the summer holidays, just after my GCSEs. I would be an extra pair of hands to help her with the charity's work, and it would give me some valuable experience for my application to vet school. I tried to be useful, but most of the time I was terrified as I accompanied her in the little van on her rounds. Although Gail's set-up was not dissimilar in appearance to Postman Pat's, she drove the vehicle more like Colin McRae in his Subaru. White-knuckled as I was, my biggest concern was actually for the rescued cats cowering in their baskets in the back. I just hoped the restraining straps were secure. Her chocolate Labrador, who travelled everywhere with her, adopted a permanent, wide-based stance to avoid falling over during the frequent hard-cornering manoeuvres.

Gail taught me a lot, and not just about high-speed cornering. She showed me how to sterilise the feeding bottles properly, how to mix up powdered milk and how to extricate the tiny, fluffy balls of kitten from the saucers of milk in which they loved to wallow during feeding time. It was later that summer that our very own newborn kitten arrived. At first, nobody knew what the flattened ball of fluff was. It had been hidden by its mother under a shed, and the wooden structure constricted its normal growth so, when the kitten was found (by a Jack Russell terrier) and retrieved (using a rake), it was round but flat, with a leg sticking out at each corner, like a quadrupedal starfish.

'What on earth *is* it?' asked my mum, who (at that time in her life) was not well acquainted with cats. Of course she knew what a cat was, but the tortoiseshell kitten was so squashed that it was not easy to identify as feline.

But it was obvious to me that this thing was a cat, even though there were certainly no indigenous mammals that looked quite like her. I also knew that she was *definitely* a she. I'd learnt from Gail, even before my veterinary training and prior to learning the basics of genetics, that all tortoiseshell cats are female because to achieve this colouration, two X chromosomes are essential. The only time that it is possible for a male cat to be tortoiseshell is in the extremely rare circumstance in which the individual is in possession of three sex chromosomes. I've only seen this very rare beast once and I took photographs of the testicles to prove it. It was before the days of smartphones, and the pharmacists in the local chemist's eyed me with suspicion when they handed me back a whole packet of glossy photos showing the external genitalia of a tortoiseshell cat.

The flattened kitten under a shed (who didn't take long to un-flatten) immediately moved in with the family, and I quickly became a cat fan. Of course, now I have treated thousands of cats and come to know and love their enigmatic ways; sometimes affectionate and purring, determined to sit on a human lap; other times indifferent to a person's emotional needs, aloof and independent; occasionally wide-eyed and wary, quicker to climb a wall than have a cuddle.

Whatever its temperament, a cat is an amazing creature. It can hide an injury or illness with skill, and sometimes its emotions too. Thirty-odd years after the serendipitous encounter with the flattened tortie, I can confirm with conviction that it is perfectly possible not just to be a 'dog man' or a 'cat man', but to be both.

Bouncing Cats

The sight of a brown cardboard box on the lap of an anxious owner in the waiting room fills a veterinary surgeon with either excitement or dread. A dog is brought to the vets on a lead and cats are usually in baskets or wire cages (although the subject of cat containers is a whole topic in itself – it is an area in which I consider myself an expert). Sometimes a lamb might appear at the practice, swaddled in towels or blankets if newly born, or sometimes, if it is bigger, shoved into a car boot, with or without straw. I've seen alpacas arrive, led into the waiting room on headcollars and lead ropes. Their presence always causes a stir. Once I even saw a miniature Mediterranean donkey emerge from the back seat of a family saloon. But a cardboard box could contain anything. If it isn't in a purpose-built pet carrier, then it may not even be a pet. Because it is impossible to see inside a cardboard box, you can only guess at what might be in it. Sometimes you can *hear* what it is, especially if it's a duck. The quacking gives it away. Hens usually stay silent in a dark box, so too owls, hedgehogs, rescued rabbits and snakes.

The contents could even be dangerous. Jim Wight, son of the famous vet Alf, aka James Herriot, recalls a story from his early days as a veterinary surgeon, when he worked alongside his father. It was the end of evening surgery and there were just two more clients waiting to be seen. One had a dog with a minor injury, possibly in need of sutures, and the other was a lady with a cardboard box on her lap.

'I'll see the dog,' declared Alf, even though it was likely to involve sedation and sutures and a good half an hour's work. 'You can see the cardboard box. I don't know what's in there, but I do know that it will have sharp claws and be dangerous!'

That observation is as accurate today as it was fifty years ago and I couldn't suppress a degree of nervousness as I called today's cardboard box into the consulting room. To increase the tension a little further, I had a camera team with me, poised and ready to capture the excitement of the grand box-opening. Laura, my producer-director, had been following me with her camera for many months, collecting interesting and sometimes amusing stories for series three of *The Yorkshire Vet*, which was rapidly achieving iconic status at Channel 5 headquarters. Both the channel and the viewers, currently approaching two million in number, were hungry for as much veterinary excitement as possible. Laura hoped that whatever emerged from the box would be either cute, unusual or both. If it was dangerous and the poor vet (me) got bitten/scratched/pooed on, then so much the better.

The box was placed on the examination table. Laura zoomed in and out on my face and then in and out on the lid of the box, keen to capture the moment of revelation as the lid was opened. Like Pandora, would I be about to release a whole series of problems? A wild bird with a wound in need of repair? Or maybe a hedgehog that had suffered a lawnmower-induced accident? The fluffy boom hovered as close as possible, to pick up any sounds from the box. The anticipation was electrifying!

'So, what have we got in here?' I asked, by way of initiating the examination. I had to start somewhere and this seemed like as good a place as any.

'I've got a box of kittens,' explained the custodian of the box. 'They are not very old. We found them under the shed and we've been watching them for more than a week. We've not seen a mother, so either she's abandoned them or she's had an accident. So, we've been feeding them with kitten food and I thought it was time to get them checked and work out if they are boys or girls.'

There was a degree of disappointment in the camera team. Kittens, while cute, would not tick so many boxes from the point of view of the programme editors. However, Laura pressed on with filming regardless, as I asked a few more questions about the kittens and their provenance.

'And are they used to being handled?' I asked finally, before preparing to make the grand opening.

'Well, not really,' came the reply. 'They've been under the shed since they were born. They're used to me because I've been feeding them, but honestly, I don't know how they'll react. They've never been in a box before and this the first time they've been to see a vet.'

'Okay, let's have a look in here then,' I said, taking a deep breath and carefully unpeeling the strips of Sellotape that were keeping the top of the box closed.

'So, what are you doing now?' asked Laura, keen for me to explain the process to our camera and possibly the viewers. It doesn't make very good telly if the main protagonist remains silent or only converses with the owner. Explaining as I go is the best way to entertain the viewer and, if it is done correctly, reduces the need for a voiceover. I'm currently filming for series ten of *The Yorkshire Vet* and I know all about this now, but back in those early days, questions from the person holding the camera were essential to prompt me and make the story flow. I duly explained that a box of rescue kittens had arrived at the practice; their mother had abandoned them and now it was time to check them over, work out their sex and approximate age and give them any appropriate treatment, such as worming or inoculations.

Now we knew the box did not contain a man-eating snake or a wild animal with a life-or-death injury, Laura and I were aware that this consultation might not make the cut, but ever the optimist, she decided to carry on filming. 'Just in case' was the phrase we always used. You never knew when a situation of jeopardy might develop.

Once the Sellotape was off I folded back the cardboard flaps, expecting to peer in and see a pile of fluffy balls of kitten, wide-eyed and blinking as light flooded into their previously dark box. What actually happened was very different. Something flew out of the box, vertically upwards as if it had been on a coiled spring. It was like a jack-in-a-box on drugs and it moved so quickly and so vertically that it was impossible to tell that it was a kitten at all. I've never seen a cat of any age move so explosively. In fact, the energetic youngster nearly hit the ceiling. I didn't have time to react to catch it and it landed on the floor some distance away, miraculously on all four of its little feet. From where I was standing, on the other side of the consulting table, it seemed okay, but the wideness of its eyes and the spikiness of its fluffy fur suggested that it was either very frightened or very surprised at the amount of elastic potential it had found in its legs. I was willing to bet that the kitten had not expected to eject itself so far. But before I could try to gather it up and inspect it for injury, there was more action from the cardboard box as more and more kittens sprang out, all vertically upwards, landing scattered across the consulting room floor. It was like a pan of popping corn without a lid on.

I looked for the camera to try to frame some sort of explanation. Alas, it was not to be. The camera was shaking uncontrollably and pointing at the floor, with Laura curled into a ball, mascara-stained tears of laughter pouring down her face. I couldn't have said anything sensible to camera in any case, because by now I, too, was bent over and crying with laughter. So was the owner! The kittens, each sitting in a different corner of the room, must have wondered what on earth was happening. One minute they were huddled quietly under a shed, the next they were in a madhouse with three humans, all crying and giggling insanely.

Eventually each ejected kitten was captured, examined and replaced in the box, and most of the tears were wiped away. The kittens were very (almost too) healthy and their adventure at the vets had, luckily, met with no injury. It might well have made an amusing story for an episode of *The Yorkshire Vet*, if only the producer-director had remained stationary!

Sandbeck's First Patient

This chapter is about a cat called Daisy. I know Daisy very well, because she is my sister's cat. She is beautiful and endearing, but not without her problems. And so is the cat. (That's a joke, by the way.) It's also about a new veterinary practice. I'll come to Daisy the cat later, but first the story of the new practice.

I am excited to report that I have recently opened a new practice. It was an opportunity that came out of the blue, when a veterinary surgery in the lovely Yorkshire market town of Wetherby unexpectedly shut its doors. It had been a small but thriving small animal practice, offering a personal service to a loyal clientele. It was then 'acquired' by a large, corporate veterinary conglomerate, swallowed up in the same way as many veterinary surgeries have been during the second decade of this new millennium.

Sadly, I suspect the conglomerate did not have the same enthusiasm for encouraging staff well-being as it had for megalomaniacal expansion. Perhaps when the final, overworked veterinary surgeon handed in her notice, buckling under the persistent burden of trying to hit targets, it proved impossible to recruit a suitable replacement and the business folded. For some reason, I was one of the first to hear about the closure and, before work one day, I drove down to investigate. Sure enough, the doors were locked and a notice was taped to the inside of the pane of glass, announcing to former clients that, regrettably, the surgery was no longer open. From the outside it looked tired and neglected, but it was still a fully functional veterinary practice and my excited mind was already hooked by its potential. My initial thoughts were that it would be an ideal branch surgery for the Boroughbridge practice where I currently worked. The building at Boroughbridge was bursting at the seams with an increasingly busy workload and some new premises could offer a solution. But the boss was not so keen. Undeterred, I did some investigation, made a few phone calls and found out who owned the building. I gave him a call. He was aghast at the news, as he had not yet been told of the closure.

But my life was already ridiculously busy. My restless mind had become hooked by writing and, in an almost compulsive fashion, I had developed an addiction that was hard to shift. Weekly newspaper columns and a series of book deals fed the habit. At the practice I was working flat out; nights and weekends on call punctuated hectic, ten-hour days. I was, as ever, in the midst of making more episodes of the ever-popular *The Yorkshire Vet*, which continued to entertain insatiable Channel 5 viewers hungry for veterinary action. I had also recently started recording a podcast, called *The Naked Vet*. The title was a nod to those occasions when I have been known to remove items of clothing before operating on cows. The podcast made a significant financial loss, but I enjoyed being creative in a new direction and it seemed like a good thing to do. Family life was increasingly complex – both our sons' sporting prowess was advancing to a national level, with Jack rowing and Archie swimming every day, and Anne flying around trying to get everyone where they needed to be, while herself working in two different surgeries. In short, it would be totally impossible to start a new practice alone. Luckily, although I don't really believe in luck as a concept, a couple of conversations offered some options and a tentative plan started to take shape in my mind.

The first conversation was with an old school mate called Mark. Mark and I had shared many adventures up icy mountains in wintery Scotland and in the soggy bogs of western Ireland. The pinnacle of our climbing and exploring escapades was on the ice caps of Iceland, just after we had completed our A levels. Near to the Arctic Circle, in the summer of 1990, we donned our crampons while we nervously awaited exam results that would eventually catapult us both to vet school. On these ice caps we felt like Shackleton, imagining that we ventured where no other humans had ever stepped. We shared a tent on these trips, and prided ourselves on having the most efficient of camping systems. Mark and I made an awesome unit of ultimate efficiency. Since then, Mark had practised as a small animal vet in West Yorkshire and helped to establish a large, highly rated practice in and around Wakefield. But now his circumstances had changed, and he was looking to relocate to a more rural part of the county and to find a new challenge. He agreed to come with me to check out the possibility of this novel veterinary business.

Late one spring evening in 2019 we met the property manager from the conglomerate. It was tipping down with rain as we made our introductions on the doorstep of the tatty premises and the meeting did not start well. The manager, who I'll call Andy, had what looked like hundreds of keys, none of which bore any resemblance to the locks on the front door. We stood hunched, sodden and cold, as Andy kept searching for the correct key.

I am a huge optimist, but after twenty minutes I was beginning to feel that our trip had been wasted. However, finally one of the keys fitted the lock and in we went. Like a newly engaged couple entering their soon-to-be first home, we gazed around the expansive waiting room, with its decor straight out of the 1980s. We looked past the empty crisp packets, bursting rubbish bins and part-drunk cups of coffee that had been neglected for long enough that they hosted exotic fungal colonies. The previous occupants had left in a rush and the lack of a final clean-up suggested a high degree of ill feeling. But, looking past the detritus, we recognised potential in abundance.

Within a couple of weeks we had a plan and a team, which involved Tracy, a practice manager with whom Mark had worked before, and Helen, a former colleague of mine. Mark knew Tracy very well and they had an excellent relationship. I would rank Helen as one of the best and most caring vets I've known. She had huge amounts of experience and had seen veterinary practice from all angles. We all shared an optimism for starting, developing and expanding a practice that was based on our combined ideals, rather than those which had been imposed upon us by the inward-looking habits of older partners or the corporate styles of the venture capital-driven multiples, whose layered management and financial targets had driven so many veterinary surgeons to despair and away from the profession in recent years. Both business models were equally depressing in different ways. This was a chance to start from scratch and make it our own.

So start from scratch we did and, in November 2019, Sandbeck Veterinary Centre opened its doors. At this point, due to other professional commitments, I was not able to practise clinically there, but I could help with the set-up process while still satisfying my other obligations. Arranging the legal agreements, sorting the finances, negotiating for the optimal computer system and helping with publicity were all things I could do. We all had our skills and our areas of capability. Helen brought her work ethic and veterinary skills; Tracy could organise and motivate with aplomb; and Mark had the vision and the attention to detail that was essential for success. I had seen this in the snowy Cairngorm mountains and during our meticulously planned camping trips. And I was just me: I hoped I'd prove my worth eventually. Our adventure started, quietly but confidently, and clients slowly started to appear.

And that is where Daisy the cat comes into the story. Daisy was one of the very first patients through the door. She and her sister, Lucy, arrived some years ago as stray kittens at the surgery where Anne was working. My sister, Kate, immediately offered to take them and the pair swiftly made themselves at home as only kittens can, climbing curtains and acquainting themselves with how to use (and sometimes how not to use) a litter tray.

As they grew older, their personalities developed and diverged. Until you get a cat, you think that one cat is much the same as the next. When you get a second cat, you quickly realise that they are all very different. It's the same with babies. Human babies, I mean. Other people's babies all look exactly the same, only some are rounder than others. Get your own baby and you realise that *your* baby is not like everyone else's baby. Then when you get another baby, the differences become even more striking. One sups milk and then calmly slips into sleep, the other screams with colic and temper. One gurgles and smiles and the other is sick on your shoulder. Yet they have pretty much exactly the same upbringing and extremely similar genetics. Explain that one.

Daisy and Lucy were just like this and couldn't have had more different personalities. Lucy was smooth-haired, active and energetic and, as she grew older, went out and hunted every day. Long-haired Daisy would rest regally on Kate's bed, either fast asleep or preening herself and scrutinising her pristine coat with bright, beautiful green eyes. Daisy would venture only as far as the food bowl or litter tray. Lucy was lithe and slim. Daisy was not. Kate loved them both, but I suspect Daisy was the favourite. As big brother and vet, I looked after them both, vaccinating them before dinner on Christmas Day or administering worming tablets during a visit for tea. It was convenient but it was not perfect because, for some reason, it is very difficult to maintain a clear, clinical judgement when treating the pet of a family member. It's hard to know why. Maybe it's because there is no computer on which to record clinical notes, or maybe the lack of an examination table. Furthermore, maybe the brother/vet takes shortcuts in explaining a clinical procedure, and maybe the family don't quite believe the chap who once persuaded his sister to buy all his unwanted *Star Wars* stickers even though she didn't like *Star Wars*. Whatever it is, treating a family member's pet is not as simple as it sounds.

Also, the cats don't like it. Yes, I know a trip to the vets might be anxiety-inducing for the pet – the dreaded cat box, a terrible car journey that might result in the emptying of the bladder or expulsion of the bowels and then having to sit in a waiting room next to a yapping terrier – but when it's over, normality is restored back at home, on the bed or in the nearby fields or next door's garden. If a vet turns up at your house, however, lulling the humans into a sense of security with Christmas presents or bottles of wine, and he sticks a needle into you when you are least expecting it, it's understandable that a cat might feel tricked and violated.

This had become the case with Lucy and Daisy. Lucy knew

how to manage the stress associated with my arrival at Kate's house. She'd usually burst through the cat flap and escape. Daisy, however, couldn't fit and, even if she had been able to, being outside would be even more stressful than being inside with me and my syringe. So, Daisy would rush as fast as possible up the stairs, with her undercarriage swaying amusingly from side to side. Then she would hide under the bed. As the years went by, a respect of sorts developed between Lucy and me, but the distrust and dislike that Daisy held for me just got worse. This was cemented when Daisy developed a peculiar skin condition. Her feet were covered in painful, oozing scabs, which required much investigation – biopsies and swabs. The solution was a series of injections, which eventually effected a cure. After that she just hated me. On one recent occasion, her irascibility reached new levels when I tried to examine her huge tummy as part of a cursory examination before her annual Christmas vaccination. She hissed so venomously that she looked like a cobra and not a cat.

As the years passed and Daisy got older, we tried to keep vet contact to a minimum. But Kate was concerned about a few issues and I suddenly had a great idea – one that would solve all the problems.

'Why not take Daisy to Sandbeck to see Helen?' I suggested. 'It's much nearer to your house and Helen is lovely.'

Both things were true, and we had specifically designed the practice to reduce stress triggers for both nervous dogs and anxious cats. The waiting room was large and airy and the colour scheme had been carefully chosen to have a calming effect – the bright and garish colours of some modern vets have been shown to be inflammatory to dogs, like the proverbial red rag to a bull. Helen arranged an appointment for Daisy and Lucy to travel to Wetherby for assessment. Lucy escaped and didn't make it as far as the cat basket, but Daisy had a great time. I sent a message to Kate later that day, asking how the first visit had been. As she was one of our very first patients, I was keen to know how she had got on. The response was vigorously positive.

A series of follow-up visits were arranged and one of these involved an appointment with Mark. Kate and Mark knew each other from our schooldays. The last time they'd seen each other was about thirty years before, probably at a party involving cheap cider, strange hairstyles, pastel cardigans and flecked, pleated trousers. The soundtrack would have been Erasure. Kate was excited to be meeting Mark after all these years and I sensed there would be some reminiscing about past exploits and old mutual friends.

When Mark and I were at school, dreaming of our perfect veterinary careers, I had always planned to work in mixed practice. But Mark once famously declared that he wanted to work with cats. Even though this wasn't particularly funny, it became something of a joke within the Norton family. At a time when many of our schoolmates could not even contemplate choosing a university course, let alone a profession, Mark had such clarity of vision that he could foresee the specific creature he would be working with in the future. It seemed prophetic that, almost exactly thirty years later, Mark was doing just that – looking after cats, and not just any cats, but the cat belonging to my sister.

The appointment went well and Mark examined and treated Daisy with his customary skill. I contacted Kate later that evening for an update.

'Do you know what?' she declared with amazement. 'My lovely little Daisy absolutely *loved* Mark. She didn't hiss or hide or anything. She was even purring!'

I was delighted at the positive news but braced myself for the inevitable comparison that was sure to follow.

'And do you know what? I think Daisy likes Mark a *lot* more than she likes you!'

I'm sure Kate was completely right about this. The skill of Mark-the-cat-vet had been prophesised years before. I would enjoy working with my old friend again, and not just because he could treat the few cats who held a passionate dislike for me! If every cat and every owner leaves the surgery as delighted as Daisy and Kate were, then the future for Sandbeck looks bright.

Smokey and the Grass Cuttings

It was quite late on a Sunday evening when the phone rang. It was also my birthday. We had already had tea and birthday cake, so it wasn't a disaster that the last remnants of my weekend on duty were disturbed. Some Sundays on call I don't get a meal with the family at all. Most Sundays I don't get cake.

'Is that the vet?' bellowed an agitated voice on the other end of the phone. 'It's Mrs Bertram here.'

'It is. How can I help this evening, Mrs Bartram?'

'Well it's my cat, Smokey. I'm REALLY worried about him. I think he's broken his leg because he hasn't moved all day. It's Mrs *Bert*ram, actually, not Bartram,' explained Mrs B., who seemed to be either quite deaf, or one of those elderly ladies who feels they need to shout down the phone because you are a long way away.

Lame cats are a common problem on all days of the week, but particularly on a Sunday. I think it is because many owners seem to scrutinise the behaviour of their pets in more detail at the weekend. Any odd behaviour that has gone unnoticed through a busy week suddenly becomes evident as people sit down for a rest on the sofa on a Sunday afternoon. Incidentally, the same is true of Christmas Day.

'Okay, I think I'll need to have a look at Smokey,' I said to Mrs Bertram, 'Can you bring him to the surgery? I can be there in about twenty minutes.'

To my surprise, instead of agreement to this sensible plan there was a shriek of laughter down the telephone, followed by a degree of outrage.

'Oh my goodness! Absolutely not! My husband and I are in our eighties! We don't drive! We haven't got a car!'

I took a deep breath.

'Right you are. Is there any way you could get a lift?' I asked cautiously. 'Maybe from a neighbour or friend? It would be really helpful if I could see Smokey at the practice. If he's very lame then I might need to X-ray him you see, to check for a fracture.'

I had been in this position many times before. Home visits to sick or injured cats, despite everyone's best intentions, are almost always a nightmare. Invariably, the examination ends up taking place under the kitchen table, or worse, behind the sofa from where the patient refuses to budge, which makes it difficult, if not impossible. It's a toss-up who gets more stressed – the vet or the cat – so seeing the cat at the clinic is vastly preferable. Often, the necessity for a home visit late on a Sunday is because the owners have been in the pub or are on the wrong side of a bottle of wine. This evening's excuse was more legitimate; but my suggestion of enlisting the help of a neighbour was met with another laugh.

'Absolutely not a chance! All my neighbours are over eighty, too. Even the ones who drive don't like driving in the dark!' shouted Mrs Bertram.

'Okay. How about a taxi?' I suggested, ever alert to a

pensioner's finances. A house visit late at night would be quite expensive and a taxi to the surgery might be cheaper. I was getting used to the response to my suggestions by now, so it didn't come as any surprise when another gale of laughter followed. This was not so much annoying as rather amusing. Already I was beginning to like this lady.

'Oh no! There's not a *chance* of a taxi in Kirk Hammerton! Absolutely not.'

There was a pause, as the cogs turned in her mind. My mind was working too – I knew Kirk Hammerton was a village just a few hundred yards off the main trunk road between York and Harrogate. Taxis would surely run along this road almost every minute, even on a Sunday. It was highly likely that a taxi would easily be able to collect an old lady and her cat.

'Tell you what. I'll see what I can organise,' conceded Mrs Bertram eventually. 'I'll go and see my neighbour Pat.'

This sounded like a good plan. Pat sounded to me (utterly without any foundation) like someone with ability and a calm confidence – as well as a driving licence and a car.

'I'll put my husband on. Talk to him while I get organised,' Mrs Bertram instructed.

Mr Bertram arrived on the phone, but not before I had gained a brief insight into the marital arrangement in the Bertram household. I could hear the conversation between the two of them in the background. It went like this:

'You speak to the vet while I organise Pat. What are you doing now?'

'I'm organising a basket for the cat' (which seemed a reasonable idea to me).

'No! You talk to the vet. He's on the phone. I've just been talking to him about the cat! I'll go and get Pat,' Mrs Bertram chastised her husband, before coming back to the phone. 'He's trying to organise a basket for the cat, would you believe! I've told him to come and talk to you. I'm going to get Pat.'

There was clattering and banging in the Bertram house as Mrs Bertram looked for her shoes and Mr Bertram continued his quest for a cat basket. Eventually, as instructed, Mr Bertram made it to the phone, slightly out of breath.

'Hello. My wife's gone to get Pat. So, Smokey. Well, he's been sitting in the garden all day. Sitting on a pile of grass cuttings. He's not right. It's definitely his back end I think. My wife, she's trying to organise a lift, from Pat, our neighbour. She has a car.'

While we awaited news on Pat and her car, Mr Bertram and I had a pleasant discussion about the other things he had been doing during the day, which had mainly been gardening jobs. Hedges had been clipped as well as lawns cut. During the brief gaps in my weekend veterinary work I, too, had mowed the lawn. It's a good job to do when on call. After a few minutes filled with gardening chit-chat Mrs Bertram returned, having successfully persuaded Pat to drive the two of them and Smokey to see me.

'Right. All good,' she reported. 'Pat can bring us to the vets. We'll see you in half an hour.'

I polished off the last slice of birthday cake – if Smokey's leg was indeed broken then I might have a long night ahead of me. The Sunday evening of a weekend on duty represents the last lap, with the chequered flag of having someone else take over the calls finally in sight. Just like running a marathon (to mix more metaphors), you can't relax too soon, because a cat with a broken leg or a cow with an oversized calf is bound to appear before (or worse, after) bedtime. But this evening's call seemed to be shaping up to be a very funny encounter, and I was looking forward to meeting everyone.

We arrived at the practice almost at the same time and I pulled under the peeling archway that led to the back of the building just as the Bertrams' transport stopped outside. I could see organised Pat, disorganised Mrs Bertram, henpecked Mr Bertram and a cat basket all struggling to exit Pat's car. I helped everyone disembark and directed them through the back door. I always do this with out-of-hours calls late in the evening. It's easier to open the back door but it also emphasises the fact that it is not a routine consultation – even something simple and straightforward takes me over an hour, travelling as I do from home and back again.

'This is Pat, who's VERY KINDLY given us a lift tonight,' bellowed Mrs Bertram. Evidently, Mrs Bertram's shouting was not just confined to her telephone conversations. 'This is Smokey,' she continued, lifting the basket to give me a closer view through the wire door. Mr Bertram, who didn't get the benefit of an introduction, stood by and watched. Smokey was placed on the table and I started my questioning again, to get a clear history of his clinical problems.

It is very important to make accurate and concise notes. Over the years, I have seen some terrible clinical notes. Before everything was computerised, it was bad handwriting that caused the most difficulty, but even now, without that excuse, some are just downright inaccurate or incomplete. I am fastidious about my own and try to record all the crucial details. Colleagues might disagree, because I have been known to make a diagnosis without much written preamble, but I do think it is vital to record accurately the client's perception of the problem. To this end, I occasionally write down in quotation marks the owner's exact words. Some recent clinical notes spring to mind, which went like this:

Reports dog very flatulent recently 'I know this because I live by myself and I know it's not me.'

192

In my view, you can't go wrong by quoting the owner's words verbatim.

On another occasion, I was presented with a crow by two people who were keeping him as a pet because he had a deformed wing and was incapable of flying. I was somewhat taken by surprise, which can be detected by reading my clinical notes of this case:

This is actually a crow. The crow has a deformed wing, but is otherwise a happy crow. Eats ham, eggs (cooked) and fried fish.

But perhaps the most memorable set of clinical notes were those written a few years ago, by a recently graduated vet, about a dog that was showing signs of apnoea. This meant that the dog intermittently stopped breathing. It is an unusual presentation and is typically seen in very fat dogs, where folds of fat can temporarily obstruct the upper airways, or in flat-faced breeds like pugs with enlarged tonsils and floppy, soft palates. However, our young colleague had clearly panicked and missed all these possibilities as differential diagnoses. In her notes she had written:

Owner says that Humphrey stops breathing at times.

So far, so good.

But then, instead of the expected list of potential causes for the breathing problem, she had concluded:

I think he keeps forgetting to breathe.

It was funny on many levels, but mainly because this tangential theory suggested that breathing was a voluntary action, considered and chosen, rather than the autonomic process we all know it to be. I hope Humphrey was sorted eventually.

But back to this evening, where it was time to focus on Smokey.

I noted down Mrs Bertram's concern, which was that *Smokey has been sitting on a pile of grass clippings all day.*

'And has he had anything to eat today?' I asked, trying to establish everything I needed to know before getting my hands on the cat.

'Not a thing has passed his lips,' Mrs Bertram declared loudly and with great certainty.

'Well he did have some of his treats this morning,' chipped in Mr B. 'I gave him some before his breakfast first thing, before I went mowing.'

This sparked another argument, along the lines of 'Well, you didn't tell me he'd eaten some biscuits!'

At this point I decided it would be wise to have a look at the patient, to try to steer the conversation away from further disagreement. I didn't want Pat, in particular, to feel uncomfortable. I opened the door to Smokey's basket and peered in. This is always interesting. Some cats step onto the table without encouragement, curious to explore outside the basket. Some burst out in a rush and leap off the table to hide behind the fridge or the bin. Some cats refuse to leave the safety of the box and have to be hoisted out. There is always a moment of fear as you reach in to grab a cat that has squashed itself at the back of its basket or box, that it will sink its teeth or claws into your hand. You can try tipping the cat out of the basket instead, but this doesn't usually work, because cats are masters at clinging on to even the smoothest surfaces, and jamming their feet behind the door to resist gravity. Luckily, Smokey, despite his apparent ailments, emerged readily from the basket. The tabby and white cat calmly surveyed the scene, before lithely leaping off the table and circumnavigating the consulting room.

'Well, would you look at that!' exclaimed Mrs Bertram. 'He hasn't moved all day long and look at him now, walking round the room! It's a miracle!'

Mr Bertram added, 'He hasn't left the pile of grass cuttings all day, but he looks fine now.'

Pat didn't make any comment at this point and I suspected she thought her neighbourly gesture had been a wasted journey. However, even though Smokey could walk freely around the room, to my trained eye he looked markedly lame on his right hind limb. I tried to pick him up, but he dodged out of reach. Luckily, four humans in a small room, even with obstacles like tables, fridges, cupboards and desks, were able to outwit the sore puss and we had him on the examination table forthwith.

I suspected either a dislocated or fractured hip or a cat bite to the back leg. The first job was to take Smokey's temperature, which is never a pleasant experience for a cat. Thermometers are the same size whether you are a cow or a kitten, so cats definitely draw the short straw. Or the straw with the widest girth, I suppose. Smokey looked unimpressed as I peered at the digital display, on which the number went up and up, past normal and only stopping when the reading was just short of a hundred and five. It looked as if Smokey would soon be smoking, he was so hot, and the reason for this was almost certainly a cat bite.

I carefully withdrew my thermometer and palpated all around his right hind limb. I found a very painful spot near the hip, with two tiny puncture holes, almost invisible but signifying where a rival cat had sunk in its teeth. The sharp canine teeth of cats are covered in nasty bacteria, which are injected deeply into the muscle when such a bite is inflicted. Almost inevitably, sepsis develops within twelve hours and, if not treated, the attacked cat becomes really poorly and then an abscess appears. I pointed out the bite to Mr and Mrs Bertram and Pat, who 'oohed', shrieked with surprise and 'aaahed' respectively. Surprised as the three onlookers obviously were that these small holes would be the reason that the otherwise boisterous tom had spent all day sitting on a pile of grass clippings, I was certain this was the cause. And if Smokey could talk, he would have confirmed that he had been feeling fine, right until the cat from over the road bit him on the bottom. After that he felt sore and poorly and the pile of grass clippings, positioned in the sunniest spot in the garden, was the comfiest and best place to spend the rest of the day. It was nothing more complicated than that.

'So, it's not broken after all?' said Mrs Bertram, before turning to her husband and spitting, 'You see, I told you it wasn't broken!'

Mr Bertram rolled his eyes. I explained that the main point was that we now knew the problem, that Smokey was really sick and *definitely* needed urgent treatment. I gave the appropriate injections, along with instructions to return the following day so that I could check his temperature and ensure he was on the mend. I turned to Pat, who had been quietly enthralled by all this unexpected cat action.

'Is that okay?' I asked, knowing that she would probably be on transport duty again. She nodded vigorously and I looked forward to another encounter with these colourful characters.

'And I'm really sorry to have spoiled your evening,' Mrs Bertram apologised as the three of them departed the surgery, inadvertently banging Smokey's box on the door frame as they went.

'No problem at all, Mrs Bertram,' I said with a smile, 'I'm glad I've been able to help.' What I really wanted to say, after the entertainment of the last hour, was, 'No problem, Mrs B. You've actually *made* my evening!'

The Cat's Bottom

Injuries to the back ends of cats are fairly common. An aggressive cat, invading a neighbouring territory in the small hours of a summer's morning at the start of an epic adventure, might start a fight. He gets bitten on the head and face as he scraps and tries to exert his dominance, like a proud male lion. A timid cat, on the other hand, runs away from an aggressive interloper. She will get bitten on the last part of her body that the aggressor can grab – near the top of the tail or on the back leg. It's a classic pattern and when the note on the waiting list says *cat, lame, right hind, off food,* experienced vets are already reaching for an injection of antibiotics and some pain relief to treat the injury.

The thing is, the long, sharp canine teeth of a cat penetrate deeply and, being as they are covered in bacteria, always inoculate a dose of *Pasteurella* deep into the tissue of a feline fighter. The small puncture wound (or two – one from the upper tooth and one from the lower; occasionally we find four tiny holes, if the grab has been a good one) seals over quickly, making a perfect environment for the bacteria to multiply. The result is the rapid development of cellulitis, which is when the tissues under the skin become swollen due to the rampaging infection. Before long, an abscess develops and the cat's temperature rises towards the top of the thermometer. The same happens to a human if the fingers get in the way of a grumpy cat. It is a workplace injury that vets and nurses dread, as it frequently necessitates a trip to the doctors, and occasionally even a stay in hospital. This is called allodynia, and is a painful syndrome where normal nerve endings become sensitised to the point that they *all* become pain sensors. Before long, and if antibiotics are not administered quickly, red septic tracts start to extend up the arm and full-blown sepsis develops. It's happened to me on a few, all too memorable, occasions; I can still recall the pain, which typically peaks at about two in the morning, of my thumb swelling and then throbbing until it was impossible to bear even the most delicate of touches to its end.

But it happens to cats more frequently. It's serious.

It was late spring and, after a morning in the consulting room, I took the opportunity to enjoy the sunshine. I was in need of some fresh air and my dog, Emmy, needed a walk. Armed with a sandwich, a dog lead and a poo bag, I set off along the banks of the River Ure. The walk was pleasant and as relaxing as the slow-flowing water of the river, and we could both have continued for much longer than my lunchtime allowed. But there was enough time to sit down for a few minutes by the lock at Milby. I ate my sandwich and watched kingfishers flashing by while Emmy rummaged in the hedge looking for adventures.

On the way back to work, we met a family – father, three children and multiple dogs – as they headed out for their own afternoon beside the river.

'Hello, Julian,' exclaimed one of the young children. The familiarity of her tone suggested that we knew each other or, at least, had met before. Since every one of the family members (except the dogs) was wearing sunglasses, I didn't recognise any of them straight away. The father lifted his sunglasses. 'It's a while since we've seen you – we are the bottom family!'

This was not much help. I couldn't think of many friends who would describe themselves as 'the bottom family'. I racked my brains; then a flicker of recognition registered somewhere in the depths of my memory. He went on, 'Princess . . . From a year or two ago. You remember, surely?'

This was the vital piece of information I needed.

'Oh, yes, of course. I didn't recognise you with all these dogs!' I said, which was a reason as genuine as the sunglasses were an excuse.

Princess was a cat who I treated late in the summer of 2017. The accident-prone feline had been out doing whatever cats do when major calamity befell her. She appeared back at home, late one evening, with the most hideous injury, extending in a large oval shape under her tail, across her back legs and all around her sensitive and important bits. At its widest point it must have been ten centimetres across. Nobody knew what had happened and I could not offer any explanation – it was an injury unlike any I had seen before. The gaping gash was truly huge and much more extensive than what could have been inflicted by a mere cat bite; could it have been a bigger creature? A badger or a fox, some of the family suggested. I wondered if Princess had jumped over a fence and caught her skin on a nail, ripping it viciously and exposing her flesh. As is often the case with cats, we would never know, but that didn't matter just now, because I had a mammoth task ahead of me.

Some years later, I learnt about the local myth, or maybe

legend, of a huge and aggressive feline that roamed the quiet streets of Boroughbridge, prowling for prey. It only emerged at night and had been spotted by just a few people. The fact that many of the spotters had recently emerged from the seventeenth-century pub, the Black Bull, hours after normal closing time, may have been a pure coincidence. Was it even a cat? Could it be a mink? Or a mutant rat, grown abnormally huge from hiding by day in the sewers and gorging on pasties fallen from the bakers? Maybe Princess had been another victim of this nocturnal nastie?

Needless to say, I took Princess straight to theatre and embarked on what turned out to be pretty epic surgery, which took me late into the night. Perineal reconstruction is a fiddly thing, because there are important tubes that need to be put back in the right place. But the surgery went well and, after an hour or so, Princess looked almost as good new – or at least, all the bits were back in the right places. There was still a question over how much damage had been done to her other internal structures and the nerves responsible for bladder and bowel control, but I was really pleased with how it had come together. I knew that when Princess woke from her anaesthetic she would be a lot happier. The third delighted person that evening was Laura, who had watched the whole thing from behind her television camera.

'Julian, that was totally amazing. Thank you for letting me film it!' she said, brimming with enthusiasm, before giving me a hug and rushing off to save the exciting footage onto a hard drive somewhere. It would be a strong story for one of the later episodes of series five of *The Yorkshire Vet.*

On this sunny afternoon by the river, as I relived with Princess's family the trauma of that heart-in-mouth evening, it seemed like a lifetime ago.

'And how is she getting on?' I asked. The last time I had seen her, the injury was healing amazingly well, as much due to the powers of the body to repair itself and the natural tendency to heal as to my painstaking suture placement, I suspected. But, having moved practices shortly after the incident, I hadn't seen Princess again and I hoped that, as well as the skin healing, her bodily functions had recovered properly.

'She's fine, completely healed and back to normal,' enthused the father. 'You'd never have known there had been a problem. We were so pleased. That reminds me – one of our dogs has a problem with his *anal* glands. We must bring him in to see you. We know you're an expert down in that department!' He emphasised the word 'anal' as if to reinforce the significance of that part of the body, which made me smile.

With that, Princess's family waved and went on their way. I walked on with Emmy along the leafy riverbank, back towards the practice where afternoon surgery was waiting for me, no doubt full of fresh anal problems. It was nice to have been recognised out of normal context, and so fondly remembered for saving the life of a family cat. Whether it was great to have been remembered for my skills with a bottom was a different question altogether!

6. Sheep and Goats

Sheep. On their fleecy surface, they are dumb and sometimes recalcitrant creatures, stubbornly resistant to any human attempt to help them. Some say they have a death wish. Certainly, they are adept at drowning themselves accidentally in the shallowest of water troughs or becoming stuck, upside down, in a hollow. In extreme weather, it is always the sheep that succumb, failing to realise that they are about to be buried in snow or swept away in a flood. They are, at times, frustrating creatures to work with. Sometimes a sheep may respond to veterinary treatment in a miraculous fashion. The effect can be Lazarus-like when a case of cerebro-cortical necrosis (when part of the already fairly numb brain loses even more function than normal) is treated promptly, but on other occasions even the swiftest and most comprehensive of treatments can prove entirely fruitless. My theory, however, is that rather than having a tendency to give up and die, sheep are remarkably resilient and that they only show signs of illness at the very end, by which time they are well beyond successful treatment. Sheep are more stoic than most people realise.

At certain times of the year, sheep are conspicuous. The noise of sheep gathered for shearing, weaning or scanning for pregnancy is hard to ignore and, of course, newborn lambs, framed by perky daffodils, provide one of the iconic images of springtime. But for most of their lives, sheep go unnoticed by most of us. They are small white specks on a green background or invisibly roaming the high fells, hefted rather than constrained by walls.

But, despite being inconspicuous at times other than lambing, sheep have shaped human history and, in particular, the fabric of Britain, not just rural life. The significance of the sheep is infinitely richer than the dozy personality of an individual ovine.

From the beginning of civilised society, sheep have played an integral role in providing clothes, meat, milk, cheese and nursery rhymes. Their movement and sales have built settlements and drovers' roads covering the length of the country in a more significant way than any Roman army ever did. One passes near my home in Thirsk, at the top of the Hambleton Hills, and is part of an ancient route from Caithness in the north of Scotland to the East Anglian fens. Cycling or walking along this track today, you can almost feel the sense of history and hear the distant bleating of driven sheep as they made their almost one-thousand-kilometre journey.

Wool was the prime reason for the development of this long-lasting relationship between man and this easy-to-domesticate species. Wool-giving sheep spread quickly from the fertile crescent of what is now the Middle East, and had soon conquered the world. Their influence extended as far as Asia, where rampaging Mongols in the high mountain plains of Siberia constructed thick rugs and tents made from wool compressed to form felt, which was light enough to be carried and so suited their nomadic lifestyle, and yet impregnable to the bitter cold of that hostile terrain. Were it not for sheep, Genghis Khan might not have been the successful and egregious conqueror he most certainly was. Centuries later, the same felt was used by Roman soldiers on shields and light armour. In non-military attire, the hat that signified a slave's freedom – a pileus – was made of the same woollen felt. Later, the British army followed suit, adopting the beret as part of its uniform. From paratroopers to shepherds in the Basque regions and freedom fighters from South America, all the way to glamorous ladies in camel coats – all these people owe their attire, whether functional or fashion, to the humble sheep and the wool it produces.

By the late thirteenth century, the British wool trade was thriving, exporting to Belgium and wealthy estates in Italy, notably those owned by the Medici family (with connections to the likes of Leonardo da Vinci, Machiavelli, Galileo et al). King Edward I sought to tap into this trade by imposing a hefty tax to help fund his fight against the French. It is thought that this wool taxation gave rise to the nursery rhyme 'Baa Baa Black Sheep'. One of the bags of wool went to the master (the king), the second went to the dame (the wool merchant) and none (in the original version of the rhyme) went to the little boy (the shepherd) who cried, rather than lived, down the lane. And think of the towns whose names derive from their connections with sheep – Skipton (sheep town), Wetherby (a wether is a castrated male sheep) and Shepton Mallet all have obvious links. So too Woolwich – a place for trading wool.

And we haven't even mentioned the powerful, water-resistant effects of lanolin, which is solely derived from sheep's wool, or the milk and cheese these amazing creatures produce, or the role that sheep played in bringing dogs into domesticated service millennia ago, or the relevance to the Scottish Clearance Act in the mid-eighteenth century – with all its implications – where people were shifted to make room for sheep. The list goes on and my conclusion is that sheep have had a greater impact on the development of modern history than any other animal. I should remember that next time I'm called out to replace a prolapse in a stubborn ewe, intent on losing its will to live. But, as the French say, *'Revenons à nos moutons'* (literally, 'return to our sheep', but figuratively 'let's get back to the subject in hand').

Prolapse!

One of the worst calamities that can befall a sheep or a cow (or any animal, for that matter, even humans – it just so happens that sheep and cows are over-represented in this department) is the prolapse of a uterus. Shortly after delivering a calf or lamb, if circumstances dictate and ligaments and connective tissues are slack, the whole uterus can evert, just like the pockets of a naughty schoolchild reprimanded by the headmaster or the owner of the corner shop for keeping conkers or lifting sweets. Until a few moments before the point of prolapse, the uterus had housed a growing calf for the last nine months, or a couple of lambs for just over five. When it prolapses, it turns inside out and will hang like either a sack of potatoes or a carrier bag of apples, purple and engorged, an impending disaster.

So when Arthur called me, late one Sunday afternoon around Easter, his pragmatic Yorkshire voice was more anxious than usual. He explained, in very plain terms, that one of his 'yows had pushed its lamb bed out'. I dropped everything and sped up to his farm in Kepwick as quickly as I could. A prolapsed uterus in any species is a proper veterinary emergency. The everted organ becomes engorged quite quickly and its surface becomes oedematous, swollen and prone to trauma and, ultimately, to bursting. It needs to be replaced very promptly. A less serious version is the condition called a vaginal prolapse, where part of the vagina and even the cervix is pushed out, resembling a large, pink grapefruit. Farmers often call this 'pushing her reed out', but I have no idea why. By contrast with a uterine prolapse, the pushing out of a reed always happens *before* lambing. As the pressure within the sheep's abdomen builds up due to the growing lambs, the weakest point gives way and the wall of the vagina bulges out. It is a problem, but less urgent and not so life-threatening, so it is important for a veterinary receptionist (and a farmer) to know whether it is a uterus or vagina that has been pushed out. Arthur was in no doubt that this prolapse was urgent; he knew it was a uterus and not a 'reed'. And what he didn't know about livestock wasn't worth knowing.

I knew Arthur well and had been treating his stock for many years. You couldn't have met a more pleasant man and he always wore a smile and a flat cap, perched at a quirky angle. His stone-built farm, nestling below some beautifully pretty hills that formed the northern edge of the North York Moors, was picturesque. He had a few Jersey cows, which he took to all the agricultural shows over the summer. They were more like pets than farm animals. I saw them occasionally, as they often succumbed to milk fever. They seemed to be more prone than most cows, producing as they did such thick and creamy milk. In more recent years he had switched from his dairy cows to a beef suckler herd, which was, at least in theory, less labour-intensive. He also had a flock of sheep, and kept some pigs for a neighbour who was short of space and time, so his farm always presented a smorgasbord of veterinary tasks. Arthur was an expert at lambing sheep, as most of our farmers were, but his old, arthritic and increasingly stiff and swollen hands struggled with some of the more complex lambings.

'I just can't get it. I'm sorry to call you out,' he would say apologetically, clearly deeply frustrated when he couldn't deliver a lamb. 'You'll probably be able to get it straight away, but I just can't, I'm really sorry to bother you.' I didn't mind. Arthur was a lovely man and, even on a busy, rushed and stressed day, he always had something kind to say. A trip to his farm, despite its long, bumpy drive, punctuated by several gates, was always a nice call.

But today there was no time to chat. The patient was half sitting, half lying down, puffing heavily through the shock of blood loss and pain. A huge, lumpy and purple uterus filled the space behind her, while two hungry newborn lambs tottered about, looking confused and frustrated as they attempted to find their mother's udder. It was partly hidden by the huge purple mass, making it hard for them to get any milk. The ewe was in no mood for suckling her new babies because she was fighting for her own life, which would come to a premature end if I couldn't replace her prolapse. One of the lambs kept standing on the delicate mucosal surface of the uterus, which could have spelt disaster, so Arthur hoisted them both over the gate and out of harm's way. It is not uncommon, when a cow suffers a uterine prolapse, for the panic-stricken animal to charge around, alarmed by the heavy viscus hanging from her back end. The uterus swings and sways and, in extreme cases, the cow can stand on it.

I remember one terrible Saturday morning, when I'd been called to see just such a case. The cow was almost impossible to handle, and the emergency had made her erratic behaviour even worse. She careered around the yard, furious and terrified. As the uterus got more and more battered and torn, I'd almost resigned myself to her imminent death. I was certain the organ would be punctured by a kicking hind foot and her insides would fall out through the hole before I'd had any chance to treat her. Luckily, we managed to lasso the wild animal and slowly wind in the long rope before it strangled her. The imminent death of not just the cow, but of the vet and farmer, had been averted. Eventually she flopped down, exhausted, and I could replace the uterus, although it was a horrible job, trying not to push my hands through what was by that time horrendously swollen and delicate tissue. Sheep, by contrast, never charge around and almost always seem to lie down as if awaiting their fate.

I remember vividly the first prolapse I ever replaced, as a young vet in my first few weeks of practice. It was late on a Sunday evening during one of my first ever weekends on duty. The weekend had been unusually quiet and I had yet to learn about the vagaries of being on call. I'd been sitting around, reading and mowing the lawn and killing time, all day, waiting in trep-idation for whatever veterinary medicine had to throw at me. Then, at half past ten, the beeper went off and it was my first cow with a prolapse. I spoke to the wife of the senior partner, who was answering the phones for me over the weekend. She was concerned – could a new vet manage to tackle this chal-lenging job? When I heard the problem, I started laughing out loud. I was delighted to be faced with such a challenge. Of course I could do it! In those days, nothing was too much. I'd had a quiet weekend and so I was ready for a big challenge. Tackled with vigour and enthusiasm, my first unaided prolapse went like clockwork – I administered epidural with aplomb, positioned the cow's legs just so to allow me to slide the uterus back into place, then put in a suture to keep it all in. It had gone like a dream.

But I was lucky – not all cases go like a dream. Sometimes, they can be an absolute nightmare. On a cold and snowy Wednesday in February, a junior colleague experienced exactly that: a complete nightmare. Without the unwavering energy and enthusiasm of the young Julian, our newest recruit, Francesca, had come unstuck with the everted uterus of a ewe. Somehow, she had managed to find a spare hand to call the practice for help and, sensing a serious problem, I was the first to respond. I rushed out, but the lanes across the Hambleton Hills were icy and it took me some time to get there. The sight that greeted me at Town End Farm was one of woe. In the far, dark corner of the lambing shed a silent farmer stood over a sheep in a pool of blood, while a shivering vet heroically held the patient's intestines in her arms. I approached, knowing the outcome would be terminal. Each breath taken by the poor ewe, recumbent and flaccid, was shallower than the last. Francesca was almost as bad, and she shook and shivered under her baggy plastic protective top. The fleecy hat on top of her head offered little protection from the chill and her teeth chattered as she tried to explain the problem. She struggled to get any useful words out through her indigo lips.

Even without her words to describe the dire situation, I could see what had happened. Small intestines spilled through her blue fingers, like long, slippery, purple sausages. The more she tried to push them back in, the more extra loops would slide out from behind. The ewe had a perforation in her genital tract, through which her intestines were spilling. Francesca had, naively, hoped this could be repaired. I'd been in this position many times before and knew it was both completely impossible and a futile challenge. Even if you managed to repair the tear, the ewe would raise her head, look around, then expire just as you placed the final suture. The size of the pool of blood and the shallowness of this ewe's breathing told me all I needed to know, and I drew up a lethal injection to stop her suffering. Francesca thanked me and shuffled, shaking with both cold and exhaustion, to the cold tap to clean her skinny, pale arms and plastic trousers. It was a gloomy afternoon with no redeeming features. A few months later, Francesca left clinical practice to work in a laboratory. I hope she wasn't scarred for life by the experience that afternoon.

But at Arthur's farm, the prolapse looked less disastrous and I hoped it would have a better outcome. There was no sign of rogue intestines spoiling the result and the uterus, though discoloured, looked intact.

'She lambed just abart half an hour ago and that just followed straight after. That's when I called, so it's not been out long,' Arthur explained. The uterus was red and swollen but not unduly engorged, nor traumatised. Admittedly its surface was covered in straw, but that was usual and to be expected and could be cleaned easily.

I gave an epidural injection to numb the area and stop the ewe pushing. It sounds technical – in humans an epidural is administered by a specialist from the anaesthesia department of the hospital – but in the veterinary world the vet is both obstetrician and anaesthetist, mainly because we have to be, but also because it is a simple thing to administer an epidural to a sheep. Mine worked a treat. Everything went floppy down in the action zone. Sometimes it's easier to replace a prolapse when a sheep is standing up, because after a certain point gravity helps pull it back down into place. If the sheep is intent on lying down, however, it is crucial to position the hind limbs pointing backward, a bit like a frog. This tilts the pelvis forward and, kneeling behind, you can rest the organ on your lap. This helps to keep it clean and stops it spilling back out as you attempt to replace it.

While Arthur was worried, he was pragmatic enough to know I could help. I'd done this and similar jobs many times before on his farm. So, as I gently wrestled with the swollen insides of his sheep, we chatted happily about how his lambing time had progressed – he had nearly finished and most of his sheep and lambs were outside, enjoying warm sun and new grass. It was a good time to be a sheep farmer and lambing time had gone well.

Eventually, after twenty minutes of casual conversation, interrupted by huffing and puffing and the occasional expletive from me when portions flowed out at the same rate that I was pushing them back in, I was starting to make progress. I did my best to hide my effort at the back end of Arthur's ewe, and soon I'd replaced the prolapse and sutured the ewe's vulva. The transformation was complete. The sheep looked completely normal again and, as I stood back to admire my work, she stood up, wobbling at first under the effects of the spinal injection, and looked for her lambs. They had well and truly found their feet while they waited on the other side of the fence. Arthur lifted them back to see their mum and, finally, they had the chance to delve underneath and find a teat. Nature is a marvellous thing and watching these two follow their natural instincts was heart-warming. Mum nuzzled at their wagging tails, just to check they were hers, and then let out a contented, low-pitched bleat.

'That's a good job,' said Arthur, offering thanks in the understated way that only a Yorkshire farmer can. 'I knew you'd get her fixed.'

I've learnt over the years that effusive praise occasionally comes from the owner of a pet dog or cat, usually after the end of their life and endorsed by a box of chocolates or a bottle of wine. Praise from farmers is never so frequent or so vigorous, but the words 'that's a good job' are sufficient to put a spring in your step.

I rinsed my wellies with the left-over water in my bucket and headed towards the car. Arthur was right. It *had* been a good job and I was satisfied with another life saved. Arthur, however, had other ideas and was not going to let me leave just yet. He was keen to get his money's worth, especially on a Sunday.

'Now, while you're here. I have another ewe. She's due to lamb any time and she's pushing her reed out. I wonder if you could just have a quick look? I wasn't going to get a vet out to it, but since you've done such a good job with that one – you've saved her life, that's for sure – you may as well have a go at this.'

And then he added, 'You never know, I might even get two for the price of one!'

I wasn't sure Arthur would get two prolapses repaired for the price of one, but there was no doubt that I had ended up with two prolapses for one visit!

Dilating in the Moonlight

It was half past eleven on a Thursday evening, at the start of a run of four nights back to back on call and the first of three weekends on duty in a row. So, when my phone rang, as I was on my way up the stairs to bed, my heart sank. When I get a call late at night, I do a quick run-through in my mind to steel myself for what might be ahead. A calving is tough, hard and physical work and this cannot be avoided. A small animal emergency is sometimes not an emergency at all and it may just be advice that is required. On the other hand, a whelping bitch who has been struggling to give birth for a couple of hours without success is likely to require an emergency Caesarean section, necessitating two hours of hard concentration and surgical precision when my brain should be asleep. For farm visits, the location of the farm and its facilities are also important factors – some of the farms we attended were forty minutes' drive away, which always made a late-night call even later.

'There's a lambing for you, Julian,' reported Jenny wearily. 'It's at Tom's at Grange Farm, so at least it's nearby for you.'

Jenny, who was a nurse at the practice, fastidiously answered the telephones most evenings. It was onerous and time-consuming work, but Jenny was committed and seemed to love it. She did an excellent job. Her evenings were invariably disrupted, but at least she didn't have to leave her sofa or vacate her bed.

I groaned and exchanged slippers for boots. Emmy, my Jack Russell, looked surprised to see me heading out of the back door so late. The clear and frosty February night was lit up by a full moon. I pulled my woolly hat down over my ears as I pondered the significance of this. It is impossible to predict whether a night on call will be busy or not, but in farming (and veterinary) folklore, a full moon is sometimes blamed for a busy night of births. I've never noticed such a pattern – many of my nights on call seem to be busy, with or without the influence of a full moon.

I arrived at the farm more quickly than Tom had expected, so there was nobody in the yard to greet me. I peered into the large lambing shed. It was full of expectant sheep, some slumbering and, despite the late hour, a few chewing on silage. It was as if they were on a cruise or an all-inclusive holiday and were taking advantage of no queue at the buffet, filling their faces and their rumens under the cover of darkness. Around the perimeter of the shed were the ewes that had already given birth, nuzzling and feeding their lambs in individual pens. Noises of contentment from the mothers and small bleats from the baby lambs as they sought reassurance that mum was nearby. But these were the only sounds on an otherwise silent night. They reinforced the maternal bond that would keep them safe after turnout to pasture when spring finally arrived.

Carrying my little bucket, lubricant bottle and lambing ropes, I went in search of the farmer, the patient and some clean water. I couldn't find any of these, so I hopped over the gate of the shed and went in. A water trough would have to suffice to fill my bucket. A generous slug of antiseptic would mitigate any risk of infection from the less-than-fresh water source. I wandered around the sheep and found one ewe in a pen, alone without a lamb. I guessed this was who I was looking for and climbed into the pen. Just at that moment, Tom appeared.

The last time I'd seen Tom was almost a year before. He had been stressed and bad-tempered because his lambing, which was drawing to a close, had been a near disaster. It had started badly with a series of spontaneous, unexpected and unwanted abortions – stillbirths and dead lambs being expelled prematurely – and had continued in just as disappointing a fashion. He had called me out to treat a ewe with a prolapse, which was terrible. Internal organs and intestines were everywhere, and all I could do to help was to perform immediate euthanasia. Tom had stomped off upset, frustrated and furious at another unexpected loss.

Tonight, I hoped I'd find the farmer in a better mood and that there would be a happier outcome.

'Good evening, Tom. Is this our patient?' I asked.

'Yes, it is,' he replied. 'Sorry – I didn't expect you so quickly, else I'd have got things ready for you! She been messing on for a few hours and I thought she'd need help. I wanted to get you now before it got too late. I didn't want to get you out of bed!'

It was a kind thought and one that does not necessarily cross the mind of all farmers. I cleaned my arms with antiseptic and applied lubricant before making my first exploration inside the ewe, who was lying down in the straw. This is the first exciting bit of a lambing, because it is when I begin to work out the details of the challenge ahead. Will it be jumbled-up lambs, with too many heads and legs all trying to come through at the same time? Is the lamb too big? Is it mal-positioned and in need of manipulation to facilitate the delivery?

But it was none of these things.

The ewe had a problem called 'ringwomb'. This is a condition whereby the cervix fails to dilate. During the normal progression of labour, the cervix – a ring of fibrous tissue that separates the vagina from the womb and which is sealed during pregnancy – relaxes and softens, allowing it to dilate so the lamb can fit through. In some cases, for no particular reason, this doesn't progress as it should and the route outwards is obstructed. Farmers usually panic, or at least worry, and call the vet. If the cervix cannot be manually opened, then a Caesarean section is the only course of action. There are various injections that are claimed to be helpful, but experienced large animal vets regard these with a high degree of scepticism. The answer to the problem of ringwomb is simple and involves time, patience, lubrication and gentle – very gentle – digital manipulation to encourage the natural opening of the stubborn cervix. I have done hundreds of these lambings over my career and the times I have failed to manually dilate the cervix are very few. Sometimes it takes half an hour or more, but with gentle persistence I've rarely failed.

I relayed my findings to Tom and made myself comfortable for the long haul, lying down on the straw and slowly wiggling my fingers inside the sheep. Progress was extremely slow, and I chatted with Tom about his lambing. It was in its early stages and, so far, everything had gone extremely well.

'That sounds better than last time?' I ventured.

'Bloody hell, yes!' Tom exclaimed. 'I was all set to pack in sheep farming after last year. It was terrible. Enzootic abortion! I'd never seen it before, but the tests were positive and I started vaccinating immediately. So far, touch wood, this year is going well.'

Tom tapped on the wooden hurdles on which he was leaning his weight. I was pleased he was in a good mood, because I would be with him for some time as I tried gradually to work my magic on his ewe. We discussed last year's lambing and this year's, making favourable comparisons. I could comment on how lambing had been in general, on other farms in Yorkshire. This is something that farmers always like to hear about. They know their own farm's experience and glean some information from other farmers at the auction market on Thursdays at the fat cattle sale, but this is often skewed by farmers understating their successes and overstating their losses. Getting information *viva voce* from a professional was fascinating for solitary farmers who were always hungry for gossip.

'We've seen an awful lot of triples so far this year,' I explained to Tom, who I could see was taking mental notes. We had already been very busy lambing sheep. Those farmers who kept sheep on the lowlands of the Vale of York, or those with early-lambing breeds like Suffolks, had already finished the stressful period. Others, like Tom, had just started the process and there were some farms, up on the high ground at the top of the dales and moors, who would not be commencing for another month or so. For vets, the lambing period lasts from early December to the end of April, with late nights and disturbed sleep for four or five months. For me, there would be many more nights like this still to come!

My progress was slow as I wiggled the tips of the fingers on my right hand into the cervix. When I pointed them like a cone, I could advance them as far as the first joint. I made the same shape with my left hand, outside of the sheep, and stared at it, assessing the diameter of the internal aperture.

'She's about that far dilated,' I gestured to Tom, making a circle with my index finger and thumb to explain my progress. Or lack of it. But there was no way of rushing this. It quickly became clear that we'd need more topics than just lambing to talk about. I shifted position so that I could lie on my back. It was more comfortable and I had a clear view of the full moon. It was very pleasant. Although this evening was frosty and cold, my right forearm was lovely and warm, at exactly the same temperature as a sheep. Now Tom and I had the time to share some humorous stories and anecdotes: I'd be here for a while yet. Tom started with a story about a young vet who had been called to lamb a sheep on his farm, many years previously. Tom's mum held the ewe at her head-end, while the young vet worked away at the back, struggling to make any progress getting the lambs out. Tom explained that he had left them to it for a while – he needed to go and feed some sheep. He returned half an hour later to see his mum still pinning the sheep to the ground and the vet still toiling away at the action end. He related how he'd asked the vet how he was getting on as he surveyed the scene from a distance. The struggling vet confirmed that he was making steady progress.

'You do know that the sheep is actually *dead*?' Tom said, having noticed that the ewe had not moved or taken any breaths during the last few minutes.

'Well, job's a bad 'un,' his mum had apparently exclaimed, letting go of the sheep, whose head had lolled onto the straw with the flop that comes with a recently deceased creature. She marched out of the shed, leaving the sorry vet alone with his arm still inside the dead animal.

Of course, with the benefit of several years having passed, the sadness of the situation had given way to a degree of amusement.

'I always think of that story when I hear a vet telling me that he's making some progress,' he added. I assured Tom he didn't need to worry. This evening's sheep was very much alive and my probing fingers had advanced another few centimetres.

It was my turn to relate an anecdote, one I'd heard from an

elderly vet, who had described an ill-tempered and impatient farmer who had once pointed a shotgun at the head of a struggling sheep as the equally struggling vet tried his best to deliver a stuck lamb.

'And he stood there, threatening that he'd shoot the sheep if I didn't get on with it!' the elderly vet explained as he told the story, before adding, 'I was just as worried that he might turn the gun on *me* if I didn't get the lamb out!' It would have been rough justice but, luckily for everyone, the lamb was delivered without the discharge of any firearm. An interesting corollary to this anecdote was that the farmer in question, many years later, actually served time at Her Majesty's pleasure, though this was nothing to do with threatening to shoot either sheep or inadequate vets.

Meanwhile, my narrowed hand was nearly inside the cervix and I was definitely making steady progress. Once it was inside, I could slowly dilate from within, more closely mimicking the natural progress of the lamb. I continued dilating; Tom continued with more stories.

'There was one vet I knew. He could lamb a sheep and calve a cow as good as anyone, and he was a dab hand with horses too, but he wasn't so clued up about dogs. He treated my dog once. He got better, but I think it was more by luck than judgement. People used to say, if he treated a dog, the first question he'd ask was "do you mind if it dies?" It hardly filled you with confidence!'

It was hard to believe, but I could imagine it, having heard similar stories of old farm vets and their ineptitude with pets. A former colleague once described the knowledge of a senior vet in the sphere of feline medicine as so insignificant that it could be 'written on the back of a postage stamp'. This was probably a little bit harsh, but I could agree with the sentiment.

Another story related to a lady whose cat was poorly and in need of an injection. The elderly vet, stubbornly clinging to clinical practice, should have retired years earlier, but refused to hang up his stethoscope. The lady, when she returned to have a follow-up check the following day, confessed: 'My cat is not much better, but that may be because the vet injected my handbag! My purse is full of this creamy, oily liquid, and it's made rather a mess, but I didn't know how to mention it without seeming rude!'

Tom found this funny and, before long, we'd passed more than half an hour sharing anecdotes about vets and their inadequacies. My hand was now well and truly inside the ewe and there was room to deliver the lamb. I knew I was nearly there and soon a pair of healthy live lambs would be born. The ewe was certainly still alive and there was no gun pointed at either the sheep or my head. I lay, still looking at the silvery moon, and I knew I had done a good job. Patience is a virtue, especially where cases of ringwomb are concerned and even in the middle of the night. It had been a lovely evening, full of *bonne humeur* and chat. All while dilating and delivering in the moonlight!

Activated Goat

It is easy to lump goats together with sheep (as I have done here). Indeed, they are very similar in some ways but in others they are completely different. Sheep and goats both come from the family *Bovidae*, which includes all the cloven-hooved ruminants, and both are in the subfamily *Caprinae*, which are the medium-sized ones. However, goats have sufficiently disparate characteristics to earn their own genus, *Capra* as opposed to *Ovis*. A goat's skin is covered with coarse, dry hair that doesn't need to be sheared every year, rather than soft, lanolin-covered wool, which does. They live in a herd rather than a flock and love steep, rugged mountain terrain. They tilt their heads when questioned, as if making an attempt to understand human conversation.

Goats, like their ovine cousins, have a long history of association with humans. Unlike sheep, they are naturally curious creatures, agile and with a great ability to climb. Indeed, they are the only ruminant that regularly climb trees, exemplifying their tendency to stray from their herd-mates and their desire to explore, pushing the boundaries of their comfort zone. Some behavioural studies have demonstrated an intelligence similar to that of dogs, which is another thing their ovine counterparts could never dream of. Even if they could dream.

I hope this short chapter gives some insight into goats, their quirky nature and endearing personalities. While I really like sheep, I absolutely LOVE goats.

It was a summer evening. I had not been home very long and I was thinking about making myself some tea. But tea was not to be because I had to respond to a message about a goat who had had eaten an inappropriate tea of its own. The message on my pager said *Pygmy goat, eaten hedge clippings.* Goats are masters of what is technically called 'dietary indiscretion'. This term, popular with veterinary school lecturers, is usually reserved for those occasions when a dog has eaten a mouldy sandwich discarded on the pavement, a long-dead rabbit or some horse poo. The result is commonly a bout of bad guts, to which the lecturers cannot ascribe a specific pathological process or infectious agent. 'Dietary indiscretion' tops the vet school list of possible causes of enteritis. In practice, we simply call it 'diarrhoea'.

Dietary indiscretion is also a very good description of goats' habit of eating hedge clippings, bushes, clothes drying on a washing line, nettles or plastic bags. The rumen of a goat has a tremendous digestive capacity, more powerful than that of a sheep or even a cow. So, my first thought upon receiving the message was that there was no cause for alarm and that I could crack on with my own diet, which was to be full of discretion. And salad. Nevertheless, I called the owner to get a few more details.

And this was when I became slightly concerned.

The story started with the 'stupid' (owner's words, not mine) husband, who had left the clippings in a pile near where the goats lived. The tale unfolded to reveal the size of the pile of clippings and the smallness of the goat, and I realised I could not simply leave the caprine rumen to do battle unassisted, especially because the clippings came from a leylandii hedge. These evil trees have terrible, spiky, needle-like leaves. I have seen their effects on the sensitive skin of cats, when they have found a dark, dry place to sleep under a leylandii hedge. I've also seen what the micro-spikes can do to the bare forearms of a novice gardener clipping such a hedge. The first and only time I have trimmed a bush with naked arms left me looking like I'd fallen in a bees' nest. I started to worry that the same micro-spikes might scarify the goat's insides, and leave a raw and damaged intestinal tract. I put my meal plans to one side and arranged to see the miniature goat as soon as it could be transported to the practice.

Within half an hour I was waiting for the patient, who duly arrived in the boot of a car. I love it when a farm-type animal arrives at the practice in a car boot. A former colleague of mine had a story of a sheep in a car to top all others.

The vet (who should rename nameless, I think) had been to treat a poorly tup that had severe pneumonia. It belonged to a farmer called Ralph. When sheep, and especially big, heavy male sheep, succumb to pneumonia, the progression can be very rapid. Fulminant pneumonia followed by septicaemia, followed by death, is not uncommon. It is one of the reasons many farmers think that sheep have an inbuilt desire to drop dead without warning.

On this occasion, just as the vet had administered what he hoped were life-saving intravenous injections, the tup sighed, gasped and then expired in a depressing heap. Ralph was temporarily disappointed but, ever the optimist, then remembered that even a dead sheep can be a useful sheep. His flock, almost inexplicably (I'll come on to this in a minute), required the annual testing of the brain of a recently expired sheep. This was a ridiculous scheme, dreamt up by someone high up in the Ministry of Agriculture, Fisheries and Food – the government agency in charge of animal health and disease control – to monitor the national flock for a disease called scrapie. Scrapie is (or, more accurately, was – it's rare nowadays) a neurological disease affecting sheep. It is caused by a peculiar protein called a prion and is connected with the genetic make-up of sheep. It is the reason why cows developed Bovine Spongiform Encephalopathy in the 1990s, when they were inadvertently fed the brains of scrapie-affected sheep.

One idea for controlling (or at least monitoring) scrapie was to analyse the brains of dead sheep. It was a daft idea. No farmer wanted scrapie to be identified on their farm, so rather than selecting the animal that was chronically wasting, scratching and walking in circles (that is, showing signs of scrapie) to be tested, they would choose one that had died of an incurable case of pneumonia or a prolapsed uterus. In short, it was not a very helpful test. So, Ralph decided to send the unfortunate sheep to the local veterinary investigation centre at Thirsk for a post-mortem on its head.

My former colleague was obviously feeling rather upset that his treatment had failed so conclusively, so he offered to take the deceased sheep to the veterinary lab himself. It wouldn't be too much trouble, as he would be driving right past on his way back to the practice. However, his car boot was full of veterinary paraphernalia and the only space available for the dead sheep was the passenger seat. The dead ram was parcelled in and belted up. He made a nice, inert and non-complaining passenger, until they arrived at the traffic lights in the centre of Thirsk. As the car stopped at the red lights, the dead sheep's head lolled forward, giving the impression it was either asleep or looking for something in the footwell. It would have made a surprising sight for anyone crossing the road. Had it been a race day, when the town centre is usually packed with racegoers, freshly out of the numerous pubs, people would surely have wondered if they'd had one drink too many. And now . . . back to the pygmy goat and the clippings.

The well-fed mini-goat arrived safely and inconspicuously in the boot and attracted no attention at all. Her name was Geraldine. The little goat did not look out of place on my consulting room table – goats love to climb on top of things to gain a better view. I conducted my examination, but failed to identify any problem at all. Geraldine looked remarkably healthy and actually rather pleased with herself. She'd managed to find some tasty hedge clippings, been for a ride in a car and now she found herself the centre of attention, standing on a table. I have come to know goats very well over recent years and find their charming, cheeky personalities quite unlike any other animals. I could tell that this little girl was enjoying her trip out. She was having fun.

One of the first goats I met, with whose character I became very familiar, was called Abby. I met her and her friends when they were just a week old. They had an appointment at the practice to have their little horn buds removed. This is an important and reasonably tricky job, and one that needs to be done when goats are young kids. It is important and tricky for a few reasons. Firstly, if the horns are not removed, they grow into huge weapons, dangerous for people and other goats. In the story of the Three Billy Goats Gruff, they used their horns against the troll who lived under the bridge. But unless you're a goat who needs to defend yourself against trolls, horns are a big nuisance. Secondly, because goats are extremely sensitive to the effects of local anaesthetic, the procedure has to be done under full general anaesthetic, which is easier and safer in a baby goat than in an adult. Thirdly, the hot iron that burns out the horn bud comes in direct contact with the thin cranium of the young goat, so caution needs to be exercised. But the eight mischievous kids, including Abby, that farmer Rodney brought to see me for their procedure were not worried. They played with carefree abandon in the room where I was doing the disbudding, weeing on the floor and sitting on top of each other. Abby was by far the most cheeky and the leader of the gang. She even chewed through the anaesthetic gas pipe at one point.

I was lucky enough to meet Abby on several occasions after this, as she took up residence on Rodney's farm as a pseudo-sheepdog. Every time I visited to lamb a sheep, Abby would appear, free range, helping Rodney and his collies. 'She thinks she's a dog that Abby does,' Rodney joked.

Ben, another farmer I know quite well, is equally besotted by goats. He has a commercial herd of a few hundred and milks them to make cheese. Even though he has so many, he treats them all as individuals. When disbudding a gang of his young kids, watching them playing together in their pens, I've heard him say, on many occasions, in his thick Yorkshire accent, 'I just LOVE goats, me.'

Geraldine, although not a baby kid, had all the endearing charm of Abby and the mischief of Ben's kids. She stood on the table confidently and healthily, but I was still anxious about the state of her insides. What, if anything, should I do? It's impossible to make a ruminant vomit, as you might with a dog who had eaten something noxious, so that was not an option. I pondered performing a rumenotomy, to remove all the offending sharp needles. This is surgery to open the rumen, thereby allowing the contents to be removed. It's the ruminant equivalent of having your stomach pumped. I once did this on a cow that had gorged herself on cow-cake, having broken into the feed store during the night. She was very sick, as toxins from the fermenting food were rapidly absorbed into her system. She couldn't stand up and death was imminent. On a cold January morning, I spent over an hour scooping out the dangerous stomach contents with my arms deep inside her rumen. Despite all the odds, that cow survived. I did not fancy doing the same on the little goat though, mainly because, on the outside, she looked so fit and well.

I decided the next best thing, avoiding the need for dangerous surgery – which would need to be under full anaesthetic – was to drench the goat with a black mixture of activated charcoal and water. The charcoal helps to coat the intestinal tract and reduce absorption of toxins. I hoped it would work, but I knew it would be very messy. Goats do not like anything being poured down their throats, let alone foul-tasting liquids, but this was the simplest option and one I hoped would help. I explained my plan and prepared Geraldine's owner, Pam, for a mess.

Preying on my mind however, was a non-clinical matter. Our hard-working team of veterinary nurses had spent the previous day scrubbing the floors of the practice with their new floor-scrubbing machine. Every trace of old, engrained blood, poo and anal-gland contents had been totally erased and the floor gleamed with cleanliness like it never had before, taking on a light lemon hue. Guiltily, I suspected that it would quickly be spoiled as, needless to say, the goat spat and struggled and tarry black liquid sprayed in all directions. It looked as if as much of the litre bottle of activated charcoal had been spread over the surface of Geraldine as was now inside her.

Half an hour later, the entire contents of the bottle were in and over the goat and also all over the floor and walls. I was not sure whether this had helped my patient, but I had certainly ruined the work of my colleagues. I bade Geraldine and Pam farewell, and Pam promised to call me with an update the following morning. My next job would be more challenging. I went to find the mop.

I'm not quite as good with a mop as I am with a goat, and my efforts successfully spread blackness to all corners of my consulting room, resulting in a terrible, indelible mess. The walls were smeared grey. At least the smaller splatters diffused more easily. It was several hours before I got home to make my tea. I'd toiled with the mop and bleach but, in the end, I needed to call at the supermarket to buy a very big bunch of flowers by way of apology to the nursing team. Thankfully, after their initial horror, they were very forgiving. A phone call the next day from Pam confirmed that Geraldine was completely fine, apart from the fact that, just like my consulting room floor and walls, she was permanently stained a deep shade of charcoal grey.

Grumpy Farmer?

Just moments after two young cats and their owner had left my consulting room, there was a knock on the door and Sarah, one of the nurses, poked her smiling face around it. It wore a hopeful expression. Her hope was that I could finish a double list of consultations in the next few minutes and then head up the dale to lamb a sheep.

The hopeful expression on the face of an overworked veterinary nurse or a stressed receptionist was one I'd got used to during my years in practice. I must have seen it a million times. When veterinary practice gets busy it is as challenging for the nurses and receptionists as it is for the vets, as they attempt to manoeuvre appointments and visits, operations and X-rays to accommodate the various veterinary emergencies that crop up to disorder the day. It is exhilarating and wearing at the same time. Sarah's notepad had the all-important instructions scribbled somewhere, amongst the telephone numbers, requests for repeat prescriptions and blood test results.

'Can you go and lamb a ewe up at Mr Whiteside's place?'

asked Sarah apologetically, 'I know you're really busy, but he asked which vets were on duty this afternoon and he only wants you to go. He says he's heard that you're the best lamber in the practice and so he says he wants you. Or Alan, but obviously he's away.' She paused for breath. 'I told him that you were consulting but he was very insistent. He says she's been on lambing for about five or six hours.'

I peered at the computer screen. I had six more appointments, followed by a put-to-sleep for an elderly dog I'd been treating over the last few weeks. Today was the sad and final day for Kite the Labrador. We'd booked a spot at the end of afternoon surgery so it would be quiet, and the procedure would be peaceful and stress-free. At least that was the plan. By now, the expression on my own face was certainly not one that conveyed any hope, because to do all these things would surely be impossible. I am good at multitasking and prioritising a busy schedule but, sadly, I haven't yet mastered the ability to be in several places at the same time.

'Okay, let me think,' I replied, mentally juggling my commitments. 'I'll just see this next one and I should be able to get there.' A colleague who was doing a minor op in theatre could be drafted in temporarily to plug the gap that I would be leaving in the consulting room. A third vet would soon be back from her horse visit. It was possible, but only just.

'And can you see if Kite and his owners could come in a bit later?' I asked Sarah. She scribbled another note on her pad, which was now as full as the next few hours of my day. Stressful as this rejigging usually is, it is a process all too common in mixed veterinary practice as routine work and emergencies collide. I remember one busy afternoon, when a whole two-hour block of consultations had to be cancelled at the last minute because a Caesarean section on a cow turned into a complex job, requiring two vets instead of one. On that afternoon, I had made my usual incision into the left flank of the belligerent cow to allow me to expose and incise the uterus, only to discover that someone had been there before, at a previous, difficult delivery. The result was an abdomen full of adhesions, with all its component parts glued together like some kind of accident in the kitchen involving a hot hob and a lot of plastic items. The uterus was fused to the rumen, which in turn was fused to the whole inner surface of the muscle of the left flank, rendering access to the calf by this surgical approach completely impossible. I needed to close my incision and move over to operate on the other side. This made things much more difficult and meant that the procedure would definitely require two vets, so I had to call for help. The operation filled the whole afternoon, and the cow tried to kick us throughout, but it went amazingly smoothly in the end, the huge calf was healthy and the farmer was happy. The same could not be said for the twelve anxious pet-owning clients whose appointments had been abolished. I hoped the accommodation of this particular afternoon's emergency would be less eventful than that one. Lambing a sheep is always easier and less time-consuming than calving a cow, so there was every chance I would be back in time for Kite.

'Where am I going, by the way?' I asked Sarah, just as I was heading out of the door. I couldn't recall having met Mr Whiteside before. I'd been at the practice in Boroughbridge for over two years and I had met most of the farming clients, but I could not bring Mr Whiteside, or his farm name, to mind.

'Oh, you'd remember him if you'd met him,' said Sarah, chuckling. 'He's grumpy all the time, his farm is falling to pieces and he's rude to everyone he meets. Apparently, his house is so dirty you wipe your feet *after* you've been inside! His farm is on the side of the hill, halfway up the dale. Turn left off the main road and it's pretty obvious, I think. It's small and messy and he only has a few sheep. We don't see him very often,' she added. 'And, according to local folklore, his woolly hat is fused to his head. Nobody has ever seen him without it!'

As I scribbled notes on a scrap of paper, I already had a mental image of both the job in store for me and also the farmer and his hat. I could imagine what Mr Whiteside would be like – I'd met plenty of similar farmers, from the old school, living alone (or maybe with their elderly mothers) and isolated from the real world. He was probably struggling to make ends meet – it doesn't take an accountant to calculate that the income from the sale of lambs from a tiny flock does not make for a lavish lifestyle.

As it turned out, the farm was easy to find, mainly because it was the only building on the left-hand side of the road for miles around. I could see it from a distance as it clung tenaciously to the side of the hill. The track was bumpy and muddy and the deep holes in it were all full of brown water, so my approach was slow. As I bounced my way ever closer to what seemed to be the most remote farm in Yorkshire, I could see my client in a dilapidated tractor attempting to move a bale of hay from one part of the farmyard to another. His progress was as slow as mine was along his potholed farm track. I paused for some moments before pulling into the yard, to allow the antediluvian tractor to finish its final turns as the bale of hay was heaved into position.

Eventually the round farmer, enveloped in many layers of jumpers, emerged from his vehicle to meet me. Sure enough, just as predicted, a woolly hat, which had once been dark blue, adorned his head, coming down past his ears and almost past his eyebrows. As Sarah had suggested, it looked like a permanent fixture and, from where I was, he looked like an exact replica of the character Benny from the budget 1970s series *Crossroads*.

It was already quite clear that the farmer in front of me was struggling to make ends meet. Even in the few minutes that I'd been there I could see that there had been very little spare cash to invest in the dilapidated farm, which was stuck in the same era as Benny's soap opera.

Mr Whiteside hobbled towards me, tottering sideways with each step. I felt for him – I was still in the recovery phase of a spinal operation to fix a worn-out part of my back. His clothes were as ancient as his woolly hat – a brown-stained, tatty pair of jeans and a thick jumper with strands of mucus from previous lambings glued to its arms, and straw clinging to and emanating from it all over. I remembered a time when I was dressed in almost exactly the same attire, during a two-week period when I was seventeen, living in a caravan on a farm in Wharfedale. I too, was lambing sheep and my hat did not leave my head for the entire freezing fortnight. My jumper did not leave my back either and, on the few occasions that I had the energy to leave the farm and head to the local pub, my odiferous outfit must have been extremely off-putting to fellow drinkers. The landlord put on a brave face but, in retrospect, having not showered for over a week, or changed out of the clothes in which I'd lambed many sheep and tended to multiple lambs, I must have stunk. But I didn't know, or realise, and I guessed Mr Whiteside didn't realise either. Or if he did, he probably didn't care.

'Hello, I'm Julian,' I called. 'Sorry I'm late. We've been busy and I came as quickly as I could. You've got a sheep to lamb?'

'She's in 'ere,' he said and wobbled in the direction of a dark yard. We both peered over a wooden gate, optimistically held together with string and faith. The building was almost completely dark and the animals inside could only be recognised as sheep by the noises they made.

'I've only got fotty, now,' Mr Whiteside explained to me in a heavy Yorkshire accent and, as if to excuse the perilously small extent of his farming enterprise, went on, 'It gets harder and harder each year. I can just abart manage with this lot and no more. I get fewer and fewer each year.'

I needed to turn my attention back to the problem in hand, knowing how pushed I was for time. The dark shed was packed with fat sheep but I couldn't see any pens or a system for handling the ewes. I'd just seen how bad the farmer was at walking and I knew the two of us would struggle to catch the ewe, even if having a lamb lodged in her pelvis slowed her movements down.

'Have you got some water?' I asked, without much expectation of a positive reply. It's a standing joke to me (although one that nobody else finds funny, except maybe a handful of older vets) that vets get presented with a clean bucket of warm water, soap (or these days antiseptic solution) and a towel only very rarely. At the start of my career this was standard practice, as seen on TV in James Herriot's *All Creatures Great and Small*. Nowadays, you're lucky if you are pointed in the direction of a cold and leaking hosepipe. And as for a bucket? Nowadays I bring my own.

As predicted, Mr Whiteside adjusted his hat, pointed into the gloomy shed and said, 'There's a watter trough in 'ere, just over thee-er.' I knew the water in the trough would be cold and I suspected it would be clean enough for ruminants to drink but in no way clean enough for performing an internal examination, yet I didn't object. Instead, I took a few steps backward and surveyed the tumbledown scene. Mr Whiteside took the hint.

'And there's a tap over thee-er. It's cold, mind.'

I grabbed my bucket and a bottle of antiseptic and headed in search of the tap, tripping over piles of debris, empty plastic cartons and heaps of plastic bags once used for wrapping silage as I went. I returned with a lovely clean supply of water, suffused with pink antiseptic, ready to lamb the ewe. The next job was to catch her.

I carefully placed my bucket out of harm's way and the two of us clambered into the dark shed. A panel of the corrugated metal sheeting that made up the roof had been either blown off by a recent storm, or deliberately removed to allow just a few photons of light into the building. It was the only source of natural light but, once inside the shed, at least it allowed me to identify the animals as sheep, which was some progress. The sheep had clearly never seen *two* people in their shed before and, it seemed, this constituted an existential crisis. It could only mean the end of the world. They ran around in hectic circles of apoplectic panic. Thankfully, the flock regained its composure fairly quickly, but we were no closer to catching our patient. I will not bore you with the details of this technical challenge, but suffice to say it lasted many minutes as the lame farmer toppled over again and again and the ewe evaded arrest. At last, I managed to dive on her in an ungainly and unprofessional fashion, whereupon Mr Whiteside flopped on top of her like a 1980s wrestler pinning an adversary to the floor of the ring. I went to collect my bucket of cold but clean water and, at last, started my examination.

This was Mr Whiteside's first lambing of the season and the ewe had been trying to give birth for most of the day. I suspected the lambs might be stillborn. The sad and premature death of lambs can be seen at any stage of the lambing season, but it is not uncommon to see a spate of dead lambs at the beginning of lambing time, which leads the farmer to despair, thinking that the same will happen to every single one of his flock. Although this never happens in reality, it is always a depressing start to the spring if the first lambs do not survive. I really hoped this was not the case today. If my initial assessment of the farm was accurate, Mr Whiteside would need as many live, healthy lambs as possible so he could pay the bills.

Luckily, the birth canal was moist and clean and free from the fetid stench of a dead lamb. I worked my hand further in and through the open cervix. I couldn't feel any feet, or a head, and I explored further. What I found was a tail, floppy and flaccid and easy to identify. This could mean only one thing – the lamb was presented in a breech position, with its backside (and tail) coming first. The back legs were flexed forward in a way that meant natural birth was impossible. I explained the problem to Mr Whiteside, who looked both comfortable and at home as he reclined on top of the sheep. He chatted amiably about his love of his sheep as I worked away to correct the mal-presentation of his first lamb.

'I sit on that and watch 'em,' he explained, pointing to a long, metal and not very comfortable-looking upturned water trough. I conjured up the image of a lonely farmer, sitting on a metal bench in the semi-dark for his evening's entertainment, finding contentment with his closest associates. I found it hard to comprehend how it was possible to get a good view of the sheep in the gloom, but I guess his eyes were used to the dim light. Maybe he didn't need to see them at all. Maybe he was happy just to be amongst them.

By now, back inside the sheep, I'd managed to unravel the back legs so they were both pointing outwards. I applied gentle traction and the lamb emerged into the world, belatedly but without problem. It was a big lamb and I was pleased to have been able to pull it out. I felt inside again for a second, which vets must always do. There was another! This one was facing forward and, though also large, it came out easily. Two large and very healthy lambs represented a good start to Mr Whiteside's lambing season. I could tell he was pleased.

I offered to help make a small pen for the mother with her new babies. It is helpful for the maternal bonding process if the family can be contained together, away from the prying eyes of other maternal ewes, who might try to steal the lambs. Mr Whiteside declined my help.

'No, it's all right, thanks. I'll leave 'em here for a bit and come back later. Give 'em chance to settle together.' He might have had visions of the sheep running amok again. He rolled off the ewe and struggled to his feet. 'That's a good job,' he added once he had regained his breath.

'I used to have a proper farm – eighty cows, two hundred sheep. I used to work all day and I loved it. Just me and me animals. There was summat in it then – you could make a bit. Not like now. I feel for the young 'uns. There's a lot of enthusiasm in the young 'uns – I see it when I go to the mart. Goodness knows why, though. I don't envy 'em, not one bit.' I sensed the old farmer wanted to talk. He went on, 'The thing with sheep is, they are all individuals.' Sounding like a character in a Monty Python film, he wanted to share some of his ovine knowledge. I was happy to listen because there is always so much knowledge an old farmer has to offer, and also because I could tell Mr Whiteside hadn't had the chance for a proper conversation for a long time.

'It's a lovely spot you've got here, Mr Whiteside,' I said as I scrubbed the tenacious lambing fluids from my raw forearms and admired the view across the gentle valley below.

'Well, it's not mine,' he explained. 'I'm a tenant – for the estate. They keep trying to persuade me to move. They'd make a fortune if it was converted to a big house. That's what's happening everywhere. That's why I'm just about the only farmer up here now.'

No wonder he hadn't got the wherewithal to make any

structural improvement to the farmhouse or its surrounding buildings. It was a common and insoluble problem for tenant farmers.

'Bang bang, bloody bang. Listen to that! Those poor bloody partridges,' he added out of the blue and changing the subject, as some shooting started nearby. 'They ship 'em in, feed 'em up and shoot the poor buggers by the hundred. It's nothing short of mass murder, the poor buggers.'

Each sitting on our own cold and slightly damp bale of hay, under the shelter of the Dutch barn, we chatted for about half an hour, touching on pretty much everything that is of interest to a sheep farmer.

'. . . And then there's your bills . . .' I sympathised but couldn't help. Small, mixed vet practices had their own financial problems too.

'. . . And how's so-and-so? Is he still, you know, having problems with his, you know, health?'

Mr Whiteside tapped his temple as if to imply it was fragile mental health that was the problem with 'so-and-so'.

'I don't think he's doing so badly,' I replied, although I didn't know any actual details.

'Of course, that sort of thing affects a lot of us, doesn't it?' said the old farmer, nodding. 'I've had my own fair share of problems, you know. It's a hard life and, you know, living by yourself, on your own all the time, with nobody to talk to. It does get you down, it does.'

My phone was vibrating again and I pulled it out of my pocket. It was the practice trying to reach me, wondering how much longer I was going to be – I guessed Kite and his owners had arrived at the practice. I'd lambed the sheep quite quickly but I had spent almost an hour talking to this lonely farmer, who wasn't grumpy, slovenly or rude. He was just alone in his small world with a creaking tractor, forty sheep and two new lambs. I'd done a good job to reposition the breech and deliver two healthy lambs, but I felt that the subsequent hour of chat and human kindness was the most helpful thing I'd done all afternoon.

7. Llamas and Alpacas

The first alpacas arrived in North Yorkshire, at least to my knowledge, around the turn of the millennium. They caused a stir in the veterinary world because nobody knew much about them. They were covered in wool and looked like leggy sheep with amusing faces perched high above – so did that mean you should treat them as you would a sheep? Reputedly, they could kick. Did that make an alpaca more like a fluffy, ill-tempered pony? They lived in a herd, so were they more like goats or even woolly mini-cows? They were categorised as camelids, so they must surely be like a camel – and goodness only knew how *they* worked on the inside! Did they ruminate like a cow? And they could spit, which no other animal known to a mixed practice vet could do. Apparently, these spits could be well aimed and possibly toxic, which presented another, novel danger. Alpacas instilled a fear of the unknown into the heart of a traditional vet in rural North Yorkshire. But they shouldn't have, because both alpacas and llamas have a long and rich history and association with humans. Their wild relative, the vucuña, from the high Andes in Peru, roamed the mountains over twelve thousand years ago and their domesticated cousins have interacted with humans – although not humans from North Yorkshire – for a thousand years.

In the aftermath of the foot-and-mouth disease crisis of 2001, during which many farmers in Thirsk lost all their animals, one former dairy farmer exchanged his culled cows for alpacas. When he turned to the practice to provide them with some veterinary care, my colleagues all took a step backward. Looking after the new herd, which comprised more than fifty alpacas, fell to me. It was a steep learning curve, but a journey I was excited to embark upon. Nowadays, I treat more alpacas and llamas than I could have ever imagined at the start of my veterinary career. I'm not an expert, but I have a great passion for them and enthusiasm gets you a long way. I quickly learnt the ways of the camelid and realised they are not at all like other animals. In fact, not only are alpacas very different from llamas – llamas are bigger, have banana-shaped ears, are stronger and more adept at carrying things and have a coarser coat, for example – but these curious creatures all have very different personalities of their own.

They have a natural curiosity, unlike sheep, for example, and they love to interact with people. Maybe it is because their huge, appealing eyes are at the same height as our faces that they engage with us more completely than many other creatures. They make unusual noises, contented squeaks and harmonic hums (especially when mating), or agitated shrills or snorts and the occasional dramatic shriek. They even make a sort of clucking noise, similar to a maternal hen anxious about her chicks and their whereabouts. They skip and dance and play by running around, leaping in a springing fashion lifting all four legs at the same time, just like a springbok. It's called pronking and they often do it just before darkness falls. I'm sure it's a measure of how happy they are.

And the mating process! To confirm how different these creatures are from other domesticated animals residing in the UK, you just need to watch the mating process. The females are induced ovulators, which means they can mate at any time and the ovulation of an egg is triggered by mating itself and the presence of semen. Performed lying down as it is, two in-love alpacas mating is one of the most tantric, serene things I've seen in a barn or a sunny field. But this is not the time or the place to discuss the sex lives of camelids. That's a different book all together.

Intensive Cria Unit

Jackie had been up all night with Ivory, her latest cria (the young of an alpaca). Ivory was just a couple of days old and, despite a problem-free birth, had suddenly taken a turn for the worse. First thing in the morning Jackie sent me a message, asking me to call at the farm to check the youngster. I knew Ivory must be poorly – Jackie was an excellent farmer and had a vast amount of experience with alpacas. She would probably already have a diagnosis and treatment plan by the time I got there, making my job very much simpler.

I gulped a few mouthfuls of coffee and grabbed a slice of toast and honey as I headed out of the kitchen door. My first job was to avoid getting honey on the steering wheel. I'd done this several times before and the stickiness always lingered for weeks. Once, having dripped honey while shovelling toast into my mouth on the way out on calls, I had decided to rinse my sticky hands with a bottle of water that had been rolling about under the passenger seat for a few days. I pulled over onto a farm track, opened the door and tipped the contents of the plastic cycling bottle all over both my hands, rubbing them vigorously. To my surprise and frustration, the bottle did not contain water at all, but sugary orange squash, which only served to make my hands even stickier. Luckily no one was around to hear me swear.

This was the last thing I needed this morning, so I shoved the last bit of toast into my mouth before setting off. And thank goodness for travel mugs filled with coffee! I drove the familiar route to Jackie's farm, contemplating what might be the problem. Crias are curious creatures, even more gangly and leggy than adult alpacas. They are robust in some ways, adept as they are at living in the high Andes and surviving in wild places at altitude, yet they are prone to illness under the wrong conditions.

Once I was on the way I called Jackie to get a bit more information.

'I'm really worried about little Ivory,' she explained. 'Everything was fine when she was born, but I don't think she can have got enough milk. She's starting to go downhill and I need her looking at, Julian.'

'I'm on my way,' I said, trying to be reassuring, 'Have you got some plasma defrosted? That might be what she needs.'

While infusing plasma might sound like something from science fiction, for a case such as Ivory it was essential. Jackie always paid great attention to every detail, and our fastidious advance planning was likely to represent the difference for the cria between life and death.

About six weeks earlier, Jackie and I had had arranged to collect blood from about seven or eight adult alpacas. This was the start of the process. Collection bags, along with reams of specific instructions, paperwork and a plastic cool-box, rather like the ones taken to summer cricket matches or picnics, arrived at the practice from the Pet Blood Bank. This is an organisation that specialises in the preparation and provision of blood and blood products for use in dogs and cats and, more recently, alpacas. I spent the best part of a day collecting blood from various willing, or sometimes not so willing, volunteers/victims. Not one of them understood the meaning of the word 'altruism'. Even for a wise alpaca, this is one concept too far. I laid everything out on a strategically placed picnic table and readied myself for the first donor, the first altruistic alpaca, who stood patiently as I clipped a large patch of fleece from his neck to expose the jugular vein. As any vet who has blood-sampled creatures that are covered in fleece knows, there is a knack to collecting blood from them, somewhat akin to the Jedi powers of Yoda and his colleagues. Sheep can be tremendously difficult to blood-sample, although fortunately for me I was taught well by the Scottish vets at the top of Caithness. There, we would sample hundreds of sheep in a morning, so I got plenty of practice.

Getting blood from an alpaca is harder still because the fleece is many times denser than sheep's wool, the skin is unexpectedly tough and the animals do not like having their heads restrained for handling. The more firmly they are held, the more they try to resist. To make matters worse, the length of an alpaca's neck means that the jugular vein has many valves to stop the blood rushing down and away from the head too rapidly, which would lead to a persistent feeling of light-headedness. If the introduced needle rests near to one of these valves, then the blood doesn't flow properly.

If all this sounds complicated, it is. Now, add in the fact that the whole process needs to be performed aseptically (so no infection gets in), that it takes several minutes for the blood to drain down the plastic tube and into the collection bag, that exactly five hundred millilitres needs to be collected (and this must be within 10 per cent, so the collection bag needs to be weighed to ensure the volume is correct), and that the bag must be agitated and mixed during the whole of the procedure, you can imagine how difficult it is to do correctly. I set about my task with trepidation and excitement, hoping my Jedi skills would be strong. Eventually, after several hours, I had a pile of blood bags, each labelled and neatly packed into the box. Where one would have expected prosecco and pork pies, I had a load of bags of camelid blood, each with paperwork connected by an elastic band. There had only been a small amount of swearing, just one alpaca had failed to cooperate at all and one bag had been wasted because the sample was too small. A special blood collection ambulance had been booked to collect everything from the practice at a given time. I expected it would have a blue flashing light on top and a dramatic legend on its side saying, 'Blood products – urgent', but it turned out to be just a normal Transit van. Forms were signed and swapped and away went my bags of blood, or rather, Jackie's alpaca blood, though I'd injected so much effort and concentration to make this work, it did feel like some of it was mine.

Two weeks later, the Pet Blood Bank had worked their magic. The blood had been separated into its component parts, leaving us with bags of fresh plasma, the liquid part of the blood, without the cells. This is full of important things like proteins, which help with clotting, but, most importantly for a baby cria that has not suckled enough colostrum, it is also jam-packed with immunoglobulins, otherwise known as antibodies. Each bag of plasma, like a bag of garden peas, can be frozen and stored in the freezer, ready to be defrosted and transfused into a baby in need. This was what I expected would be required this morning, to give Ivory a big and very specific boost.

When I arrived Jackie was obviously worried, but was ready

for action. She had already begun the plasma-defrosting process, which cannot be hurried in the microwave for fear of damaging the delicate proteins. I examined Ivory. While she did not look close to death's door, she was lacking the usual vitality of an energetic youngster. It can be helpful to perform blood tests at this point, to check how much colostrum has been taken in. Colostrum, the first antibody-rich milk that comes from the mother, provides all the maternal protection that is needed for a baby in its first days and weeks. But analysing Ivory's blood would only delay her treatment and it is generally accepted that the sooner the immunity is boosted the better. I gathered everything I'd need and made my preparations. If collecting blood from an adult alpaca had been hard, this next stage would be even more challenging. Ivory was no bigger than a small dog and her jugular vein was thinner than a thin pencil. I needed to place an intravenous catheter, keep it in place and keep her still for twenty minutes while all the life-preserving plasma went where it needed to go. Inwardly, I cursed myself for not asking Jackie to bring Ivory into the practice, where nurses, drip stands, bandages and tape would be at our disposal to make the procedure easier. It would be much harder in a barn.

Jackie sat in a chair with Ivory on her knee while I clipped the curly fleece. Luckily, there was a conveniently placed hook from which I could hang the bag of plasma. I attached the giving set. This is the long, plastic tube that takes fluid from the bag to the patient. A special one is needed for this sort of infusion, with a fine filter to ensure no tiny clots go through. Everything was ready and I drew a deep breath before inserting the cannula. I was lucky. It slid in first time and dark blood issued from the open end. The next stages I could do in my sleep and it didn't make any difference whether the patient was an alpaca, a cat or a horse. Soon, everything was attached and the plasma ran in steadily, drip by drip. To rush the fluid in is dangerous and can result in a dramatic anaphylactic reaction, characterised by swelling of the face and strange noises, so caution was really critical.

But there was no facial swelling and Ivory didn't make a sound, strange or otherwise. The barn made a more than adequate intensive care unit and the procedure went spectacularly smoothly. Almost miraculously, once we had detached her from the drip, Ivory skipped back to her mum as if nothing had happened. Were my eyes tricking me or did she look better already?

This was the first plasma transfusion we had carried out on a baby alpaca and it had gone extremely well. Both Jackie and I felt certain that it had saved Ivory. The planning had paid off, as meticulous preparations usually do. And even better, next to the frozen peas in Jackie's freezer there were more bags of plasma. I'd learnt a new trick and one that I hoped might be crucial for saving more lives in the future.

It wasn't long before another bag of plasma was needed for another baby on another farm. Noah was a baby llama, just five days old. At first he had thrived under the close supervision of his proud mum, Anya, and had seemed to have enjoyed a great early start; but suddenly things took a turn for the worse. Noah suddenly stopped skipping and playing. His *joie de vivre* evaporated. He tried tirelessly to suck sustenance from his mother's teats, but still he deteriorated. Diligent care from Suzanne, his owner, quickly identified the problem. Anya's milk had changed to something more akin to the glue that children use to stick glitter onto paper. Thick and gooey, it lacked any volume or nutritional value and Noah's previous good health slid downhill rapidly. One morning, his head, petite as it was, proved too heavy for his delicate neck to support and he lay down, inert, on the straw bed of the barn that had been his home so far. He was weak, cold and plunging rapidly towards death.

Frantic phone calls followed, the result of which was a llama trek to the practice, with a bag of plasma slowly warming in the glove compartment of Suzanne's car and a newborn llama strapped into the passenger seat. Meanwhile, we readied ourselves for this unusual patient, preparing everything we would need for the infusion. Clippers, catheters and bandages were all lined up, along with syringes of antibiotic, the glucometer to measure blood glucose and the fluid administration set. It was much easier to create a slick ICU (Intensive Cria Unit) in the clinical setting of the practice than it had been in a straw barn. When Noah arrived, it was a bit like a scene from the American hospital drama series *ER*. Noah (who coincidentally shared his name with Noah Wyle, the actor who played Dr Carter in the afore-mentioned TV show) was rushed into theatre and we set about prepping him to be infused with the same life-enhancing elixir that had worked so well for Ivory. In fact, the fluid Noah was about to receive had been donated by an alpaca, but the creatures are similar enough for this to be not only possible but also safe.

Noah's temperature was so low that it didn't register on the thermometer. This was a terrible sign, but not an indication of neglect or hypothermia through exposure; rather, it represented circulatory collapse – his little body was shutting down. Noah's blood glucose measured just two. It should have been six. He was dying. We had a conflab and gave him a 20 per cent chance of survival.

But these creatures are designed to survive in rougher places than North Yorkshire. The altitude of the Andes and the chal-lenges that life in the high mountains bring make llamas more robust, rugged and more determined than their cute, thoughtful faces suggest. As the plasma ran into Noah's vein, it was almost possible to see the life returning to his limp body. Sugary solu-tions were applied to his cold gums, intravenous antibiotics were instilled to fight any risk of infection overwhelming his weak immune system and we wrapped him in bubble-wrap and blankets. By the time the plasma had run in, Noah was able to hold his head up – no mean feat, since his neck was so long and had been so floppy. We added a bag of glucose-rich fluid next to continue to boost his system. By teatime he could stand and by evening he was travelling back to the farm, still attached to his drip. Suzanne was thoroughly briefed about how to monitor the catheter and giving set to ensure the fluid dripped into his vein continuously. Even though it would be hard to manage intensive treatment back on the farm, everyone was acutely aware that Noah stood his best chance with Anya, his doting mum, watching over him.

I was on duty the next day, a Sunday, and I made the trip across the moors to check on Noah. Suzanne looked exhausted – she'd been up with him all night.

'I feel like an intensive care nurse,' she told me, stifling a yawn. Noah, on the other hand, looked chipper. With encouragement, he could stand up and totter about. I checked his temperature – it had risen by around ten degrees on the centigrade scale and was now normal, which was remarkable. I checked him over and could tell he was on the mend. He was by no means out of the woods yet, but he could see the light coming through the leaves of the clearing ahead. I took some blood to check his glucose. It had risen to just over four and a half, which was almost normal! He wobbled round to Anya's underside, poking his head between her back legs, looking for a meal, but it was clear that there was precious little milk emanating from her teats, just the gluey white stuff from before. He wouldn't suckle from a bottle either. But it was crucial that he get oral sustenance somehow. He couldn't live on intravenous therapy for long. I reached for my trusty lamb feeding tube – a soft, flexible tube that had provided life-saving nutrition for countless lambs over the years. I slid it gently to the back of his mouth, using my thumb to stop him chewing on the pipe. The last thing I wanted was for it to be bitten in half and then swallowed. It's essential that the tube enters the oesophagus and not the windpipe, and care must be taken as it is gently advanced. The head must be held in a natural, neutral position and not extended. Once in, there should be gentle attempts at chewing rather than the vigorous reflex of excessive coughing that quickly happens if the tube, like a hastily swallowed drink, goes down the wrong way.

But there were no disasters with the tubing and it all went to plan. Moments later Noah stood up, unassisted, and squatted to pass a long stream of clear urine. It was a small victory, but brought huge smiles to my and Suzanne's faces. It looked like another life had been saved by the magic plasma. That, and a lot of hard work!

Alpacas in the Practice

After Noah's successful trip to the practice and his amazing recovery thereafter at home on the farm, there seemed to be a steady stream of camelids appearing at the surgery for treatment. Not only was it eminently possible to bring these fluffy creatures to the clinic – they were, after all, much more portable than a heifer or a horse, for example – but their inquisitive nature made it seem as if they actually enjoyed the trip out.

Fido, although he had a name more traditionally attached to a dog, was an alpaca, and he had a retained testicle. I'd discovered it, or the lack of it, during the routine examination of a group of young males prior to their castration. Male alpacas and llamas are extremely driven by hormonal urges and have a voracious appetite for sex. In part, this is because females are sexually responsive all year round. Most other animals come into season, more correctly known as oestrus, at specific times – cows, for example, every three weeks and bitches usually twice a year – and mating is only possible at these set times. A female alpaca is ready and willing (and usually very keen) to mate at all times, except when she is pregnant. It's a great evolutionary adaption to improve fertility and conception. The result of this is that male alpacas are in a constant state of sexual arousal. Most domestic alpacas are small groups of males because the majority of pet owners do not have the skills or capacity to keep males and females together. If they did, two or three alpacas would quickly turn into a breeding herd. If males in a group are left entire, the results are akin to what might happen on a Friday night in a busy city centre, before or after a trip to a nightclub – testosterone-fuelled young males all ending up strutting their stuff, antagonising one another and vying for the top position. Fighting will ensue and the consequences can be disastrous.

Male alpacas are almost designed for fighting; they have long, curved teeth like scimitars. To reinforce what they see as the masculine hierarchy, they use these hooked teeth to bite the testicles of their rivals, obviously not a very nice thing to do (incidentally, fighting male rabbits do the same thing). Castrating the males removes the testosterone-related urge to fight and this antisocial behaviour is quickly stopped in its tracks. So, unless you happen to be a stud male, which is the best job an alpaca or llama can have, a male alpaca or llama will always need to be castrated so he can't damage his friends.

Fido's missing testicle was a problem. All his friends had two, nestling snugly in their scrotums, and they do nestle snugly, held tightly against the perineum and below the anus. (They don't dangle like in a large dog or like a bull's testicles, which hang so low they can sometimes be stood on!) They were easily and swiftly removed. Fido had only one in his scrotum, which meant the other one had not properly descended and stubbornly resided in his abdominal cavity. If it was left there, it would continue to produce testosterone and havoc would be wrought, even though the others alpacas were all castrated.

We pondered the options, the best one of which seemed to be to perform exploratory surgery under general anaesthetic in the clinical setting of the practice. I'd done the same thing recently on a miniature donkey and it had worked a treat. An adult male alpaca is large, but not much bigger than a Great Dane or Irish Wolfhound, so I felt sure there would be enough space in the operating theatre.

We arranged a day and, when it arrived, kept the waiting room quiet as Fido arrived, with three friends to keep him company and reduce his stress levels. Alpacas and llamas, despite their testosterone-induced arguments, form very strong bonds with one another. They all have their own special friends. Fido's bestie, who stood closely by his side in the unfamiliar surroundings of the veterinary surgery, was Lothario. Lothario had achieved fame of his own as a stud male and as an early star of *The Yorkshire Vet*, when I performed a fertility test on the supposedly virile youngster. While his early breeding career had been illustrious, latterly it had not been so successful and my test revealed that he had become infertile. His retirement was well deserved and it was hoped that he and Fido would enjoy their later years together, free from the hassles and challenges of the competition for females.

I can still remember the heads turning as four fluffy creatures, each one as tall as a person and with mad frizzy hair, calmly walked into the waiting room and waited their turn to be seen. They looked like a four-piece rock band from the 1980s.

The operation went smoothly and before long the fab four were on their way home to start the rest of their almost well-behaved, fight-free lives.

Hope, a young cria, waited patiently in the waiting room accompanied, like a child at the dentist, by her mum. She'd had an ongoing problem with a swelling on her front leg since she was a week or so old and it wasn't improving. It appeared to be something called an angular limb deformity, which is a grand way of saying that she had a bent leg. Because of the ridiculous length of a camelid's legs, even a slight abnormality in alignment or orientation can cause a dramatic deviation. Left unaddressed and over time, this can get worse rather than better. Hope skipped and pronked without any obvious pain, but the time had come for further investigations and I had arranged for the youngster to have some X-rays taken. This is a common thing to do with a dog or cat, where the sedated patient lies perfectly still and properly positioned to get superbly detailed images. But I didn't really want to sedate Hope, so I decided to deconstruct the radiography machine, unscrewing the headpiece so it could be positioned on its side, resting on the floor. Rather than taking a view from above, I could take the X-ray horizontally, with Hope standing quietly next to her mum. They both looked calmly around the radiography suite (I call it a suite, but it's actually just a room), apparently curious about all the equipment and paraphernalia, as I lined up the beam. Just as curious as Hope and her mum, nurses and vets appeared from all corners of the practice to witness the occasion of a young alpaca being X-rayed. Would it work? Would the images be diagnostic? Or was this another of Julian's hare-brained ideas that might yield nothing useful?

I clicked the button and fed the cassette into the processor. With this machine, as if by magic, the digital processor sucks the picture from an A4-sized, hard plastic cassette, and an image in black and white and various shades of grey appears on a computer screen. I'm old enough to know that this is *actually* magic because, at the start of my veterinary career, we used to make these images come to life by dipping rectangles of celluloid into pungent chemicals that rotted the cuffs of your woolly jumper. If the stars were lined up correctly and if we said a prayer to Agfa, the god of photographic processing, an image would develop. If we remembered to dip it in the fixing solution, it wouldn't disappear and fade, via sepia, into blurred obscurity.

With Hope (and I mean the alpaca rather than the emotion), the magic of digital processing eventually yielded a set of X-rays on the screen in front of me. Everyone peered at the images, expecting, I suspect, to see that my alpaca's trip to the practice had been a complete waste of time. In fact, the diagnosis was there before our eyes. The distorted swelling and irregular bony pattern just above Hope's carpal joint demonstrated a clear case of epiphysitis. This prompted oohs and aaahs from the onlookers, amazed that my efforts had yielded both a diagnosis and also a fantastic word. Complicated as this word sounds, like most things it's not as mysterious as it might seem. A rule that all medical and veterinary students learn on the first day at university is that anything ending in -itis means 'inflammation of'. The thing that is inflamed is the bit before the -itis. So, epiphysitis simply means 'inflammation of the epiphysis'. The epiphysis is the end part of a long bone and the bit from where growth emanates. In animals like alpacas, lambs and cattle, this growing area can be prone to any infection that may creep into the body via the navel, shortly after birth. If infection settles in a joint, the result is 'joint ill' – a septic arthritis, which is much more common.

I'd never diagnosed epiphysitis on an X-ray before – mainly because I hardly ever X-ray a lamb or a calf. Today, Hope had given me the chance to establish a proper and definitive diagnosis using modern methods. This was a good example of a case that could move veterinary medicine forward. You would rarely find a farmer who would volunteer a lamb to have its leg radiographed – it would be far too expensive, and anyway a presumptive diagnosis would usually suffice. It is one of the best things about treating alpacas and llamas. Whether it's taking an X-ray to facilitate a proper diagnosis or transfusing plasma to cure a life-threatening illness, the opportunity to delve deep into veterinary medicine makes working with these species extremely rewarding. It's because their owners are so devoted.

Hope's treatment involved a prolonged course of antibiotics to penetrate the affected area of bone and cartilage and kill the infection. After four weeks I called in to see her, back in her field with mum. She scampered around at high speed with barely a trace of lameness and a leg that was almost perfectly straight.

Some months later, I found myself examining another young alpaca with bent legs. Olivia was her pretty name and it was apt, for she was a very beautiful alpaca. She was just a few weeks old and, in contrast to Hope, who only had one bent leg, Olivia was as bandy as a Queen Anne chair, with her front legs flared outwards. She was struggling to stand up and, quite rightly, her owner Doug was becoming anxious. Initially, we hoped that the deviation, known as carpal valgus, would correct itself. (The opposite condition to valgus deformity is called varus, where the legs point inwards. As a student it was easy to remember which was which, because it was vulgar to have one's legs pointing outwards. That's what the lecturers told us anyway.)

Some deformities do correct themselves, without any intervention. Young bones are soft and change considerably as the body grows. This allows ample scope for correction to occur. But it can also open the door for the defect to worsen, and this was my fear for Olivia. Each time she struggled to get to her feet, the outward buckling seemed to get worse. The solution, I thought (or hoped), was a splint on each leg.

I'd met Olivia before. In fact, my face was the second one she'd ever seen, as I had delivered her – amidst something of a crisis – on a warm summer evening. It was a peculiar scene. In a field, a white adult alpaca was sitting down. Out of her rear end stuck the smaller head of a yet-to-be-born cria. Doug had called in a panic and I'd dropped everything and rushed to help. Olivia's mini-head was looking around, quite calm but obviously wondering if there was more to life than this. As my lubricated hand explored alongside Olivia's head, the cause of the problem became clear. Both front legs were flexed at the carpal joint, pointing back inside rather than arranged in the streamlined position crucial for a simple birth. Gently, I extended one leg, then the other, and Olivia was quickly out. At this point, of course, it was not apparent that the bent legs that had contributed to the difficult birth would bring other problems in just a few weeks' time.

The day I was to have my second meeting with Olivia I had a couple of spare appointments before the start of evening surgery. 'Can you bring her down, Doug?' I asked, mindful that I'd need plenty of bandage material. I was not yet sure exactly how I would proceed. It might require splints, or just sturdy support bandages. Maybe she'd need a pair of casts? I'd be able to do a much better job in the practice, where there was a cupboard full of bandaging equipment, rather than using just the basics in my car boot. I offered the twenty-minute free period in my afternoon, and Doug jumped at the chance. 'Yep, I'll see you in half an hour,' he confirmed in his typically cheerful manner.

Olivia was the third alpaca to come to the practice in as many months. This was getting to be a habit. Once, the sight of a camelid in the waiting room caused surprised looks, but now it was becoming commonplace. To see a fluffy face peering over the reception desk had quickly become the new normal.

Olivia wobbled around the waiting room, dodging dogs and tripping over cat baskets like the disorientated giraffe in the film *Madagascar*. Her long, deformed legs did not agree with the slippery surface of the waiting room floor. It's an irksome design fault of veterinary practice floors that the requirements for efficacious hygiene and confidence-inducing underfoot grip do not align. Doug quickly realised it was much easier for all concerned if Olivia was carried into my consulting room. I made my acquaintance (I don't think Olivia recognised me from our first encounter) and then set about palpating her limbs, quickly discovering a marked laxity. The carpal joint – the equivalent of our wrists – could be easily moved outwards. This was surely a congenital defect – possibly triggered by the abnormal birth, or maybe the cause. I was fairly sure that it should rectify itself as the ligaments around the joints strengthened with maturity and movement. However, every time the unfortunate cria put her full weight on the legs the deviation was exacerbated, so I felt sure some supporting splints would provide the answer. I explained my plan to Doug, who was happy to go ahead.

I collected a box of bandages and got to work, wrapping Olivia's legs up in two elbow-long blue and stiff supporting splints that looked like the legwarmers worn by dancers. They looked mighty effective, I had to say, and I stood back proudly to admire the rigidity of my structures. But there was a flaw in my plan. Olivia's front legs were so long and so rigid that she couldn't get herself onto her feet!

Doug and I scratched our heads. Maybe we should concentrate on fixing one leg at a time? I carefully lifted Olivia to her feet. Despite the slippery surface, once she was up she acquitted herself quite well, and quickly proved that even though she couldn't really walk, at least she could totter. She looked like a little girl trying to walk in her mother's high heels.

'The thing is, Doug, I think she'll only need them on for a week or so, just to let the ligaments stiffen up,' I explained, in an attempt to lighten the mood. Doug nodded doubtfully as he carried her to the car and made her comfortable on the front passenger seat. The little cria had enjoyed more drama than most in the few weeks of her short life. I fastened her seat belt safely around her chest and neck. After all, we didn't want any more accidents with Olivia!

Alpacas on the Telly

My experiences with Olivia and Noah proved that it was simple to treat an alpaca or llama in a clinic situation. Moreover, as Olivia pranced around the waiting room, showing off her new kinky boots, it seemed that they really did love getting off the farm, apparently relishing social interaction. It was as if they actually enjoyed showing off!

So, when I got a call from the producers of *This Morning*, ITV's daytime chat show presented by Holly Willoughby and my childhood hero Phillip Schofield, asking me to appear and to take some sort of animal along with me, alpacas were the obvious choice. They were not afraid to explore the boundaries of their comfort zone, and experience had shown me that they liked the attention.

Once upon a time I would have run a mile if asked to appear on live television. But, as a result of my ongoing involvement in *The Yorkshire Vet* series, there didn't seem to be such a thing as a comfort zone any more and, increasingly, I found myself agreeing to do all sorts of things that would once have filled me with dread. Appearing as a guest on *This Morning* would certainly be a far cry from my usual veterinary antics in Yorkshire, where my only audience was a farmer or the owner of a cat, dog, horse or pig.

But, as usual, I found myself jumping in with both feet. 'I'm sure I can find an alpaca or two. They'd make great guests!' I found myself volunteering, before adding, 'And I can link it to the story in my book that featured an alpaca sex clinic.' I was fully aware that the reason for going on the show was to promote my latest book. I was also fully aware that this topic was bound to raise both Holly's eyebrows and a smile!

The alpacas took some arranging. Luckily, I have a few good friends in the camelid world with useful connections. Also lucky was the fact that people in the world of alpacas are hugely passionate and energetic about the species they love. I felt sure I could find someone not too far from London who was as evangelical about alpacas as I was, and before long and after only about ten emails, I managed to find a well-behaved and local pair ready to go, along with their owners, to Television Centre, Wood Lane, London. I recognised the address because it was the same one that I used to write to when I entered a *Blue Peter* competition, or to where I would send collected stamps or milk bottle tops for an appeal to save something or help someone. But that was when I was ten years old. Now I was in my forties, but I was just as excited!

And so it was that, on a Thursday morning in February, Spitfire and Pete the alpacas and I arrived at the 'talent' entrance of this famous place. Spitfire was friendly and composed, but somewhat aloof. Pete and I, however, hit it off like a pair of kindred spirits. As the friendly alpaca and I chatted and made friends in advance of our live TV debut, I suspected there might be pandemonium on set before too long.

The alpacas went first, for an introduction to the TV presenters and to benefit from a rehearsal. I didn't get to rehearse and I'm not sure why. Did they think I was a live TV pro? And why would animals need a rehearsal anyway? I was confused and slightly apprehensive. My lack of rehearsal did not matter though, because it was not me that took centre stage. My new bestie Pete the alpaca took that honour.

Within minutes of the animals meeting Holly and Phillip, tension developed. Holly is notoriously nervous around animals (they had had a pig on the previous day and he had caused havoc) and she stayed at a safe distance. Phillip, for his part, was not nervous but, despite his role as Dr Dolittle in the West End production, was evidently reasonably inept around animals. He pulled on the alpacas' lead ropes as Holly observed from afar. Pete sensed the unease – lead ropes need to be held gently and pulling only causes a confrontation. And confrontation there most certainly was. Pete spat directly into the multi-award-winning presenter's face, causing much amusement to the production team. Holly, not for the first time, collapsed on the floor in a fit of helpless giggles.

Thankfully, composure was soon regained by all. Phillip wiped the spit from his face and Pete calmed down. Minutes later, I was called into action, holding onto the alpacas and acting as referee. We talked, live on national telly, as naturally as if we were standing waiting for a bus or having a drink in the pub – me, a Yorkshire vet, looking after two alpacas, along with possibly the two most famous telly presenters of recent times. I had to pinch myself because it was hard to believe.

But the glamorous world of green rooms and celebs would be short-lived. Later that day, after a return journey north, I would be back in proper veterinary action and on call again. It would be familiar territory, firmly within my area of expertise.

That said, the world of telly is a novel and exciting one. It's even better with a couple of alpacas by your side!

Camelid Calamities

'It's Cinderella, Julian. She's started lying around in odd places and pushing a bit, but something's not right. Can you come and have a look?' Jackie asked, in a calm but urgent conversation on a Tuesday lunchtime.

Not many clients have my mobile phone number. Some vets see divulging their number as a dangerous thing to do. It means you are never free from calls and always on hand. But Jackie had my number more as a friend than a client, and she only ever called or messaged when it was an emergency. Today's call had the potential to be just that.

As chance would have it, I was on a house call to vaccinate a dog belonging to a couple who were housebound and I was only fifteen minutes away from Jackie's farm and Cinderella the alpaca with her un-progressing, first-stage labour. Dealing with the dog was a simple affair, and I was quickly en route and contemplating what might be in store for me when I arrived at the farm.

This is one of the best things about being a vet in mixed

practice. Yes, it's stressful at times – busy and unpredictable, with high-pressure situations appearing out of the blue (such as today) and at inconvenient times on a daily basis. While I was rushing at speed along the winding lanes to see Cinderella, I should have been heading for a quick bite of lunch before following up a series of ongoing cases during afternoon surgery. As on many other occasions, my afternoon would need to be rearranged. But, once you've accepted the inevitability of another hungry afternoon haphazardly altered by an emergency visit, and after the apologetic phone calls have been made, excitement replaces the annoyance of the unexpected change of plan. The journey to a call like this is very exciting, as I run through in my mind all the possible things that I might encounter when I arrive. Today was no exception. In fact, my anticipation was near an all-time high.

Usually, alpacas give birth without any problems at all and they almost always have a single cria. Twin pregnancies are very rare, so there is almost zero chance that two babies will get tangled up, which is often the case with lambs. It's also extremely rare that the cria is too large, which can be a common cause of problems in cattle. Cinderella and I had history because she'd presented me with one of the most difficult deliveries I had ever done when she had given birth three years earlier. When I arrived on that occasion, Cinderella had looked as forlorn as her pantomime namesake when she thought she'd be missing out on an evening at the ball. She was clearly in some distress, which was not surprising because she was trying to deliver a cria in the breech presentation. This is where the baby is trying to come out bottom first. The back legs are bent forward and need to be flipped round so that both are pointing backward to allow delivery. Because an alpaca's legs are so very long – like every other part of an alpaca – it was really difficult to straighten the legs to allow the birth to be possible. Somehow, I'd eventually managed to get things sorted out and a very lively little cria eventually emerged, looking rather like E.T., into the world. Surely, I pondered, as I drove along the lanes towards the farm, she wouldn't have the same problem again? Lightning couldn't strike twice, could it?

It wasn't that camelids were particularly prone to calamities – in fact usually it's quite the contrary; llamas and alpacas are generally robust and tough, and are extremely easy to look after. But I had recently been called to treat a few catastrophes. There was the time when three young alpacas had broken into the feed bin during the night and gorged themselves on tasty food. The result was three alpacas with choke and another urgent call. Choke is an upsetting condition, which can be fatal if not addressed quickly. On that stressful morning, I found myself passing stomach tubes, instilling fluids and even holding the youngsters upside down to encourage the chomped-up food to come out the way it went in.

Then there was the time recently when another of Jackie's alpacas had prolapsed her uterus shortly after giving birth. The red, rugby-ball-shaped and -sized uterus protruding angrily told a story of urgency all by itself.

On another occasion, I rushed to see a llama called Gus at a trekking centre. Gus was choking and in a very bad way. Upon examination, it became clear the obstruction was an immoveable mass and I suspected the elderly llama was suffering from a tumour in the oesophagus. This is more common than you might imagine, often because of the ingestion of bracken – strictly off the normal menu but easy to grab by the mouthful when out trekking – which can cause cancerous changes in the gastrointestinal system. I'd seen a handful of similar cases over the years

I had been dealing with llamas. Gus had, apparently, loved to nibble on this potentially dangerous plant more than most. It was clear that a rapid solution to his suffering was required. Accompanied by many tears, the final injection went in smoothly and the heroic old llama slipped peacefully off to sleep.

It went so smoothly, in fact, that Dave, Gus's owner, did not even notice that I'd given the jab. 'He's beaten you to it, Julian,' Dave whispered from where he was sitting on the llama's opposite side, stroking his old friend's neck.

'No, that's my injection,' I replied. 'It's just gone in. It works pretty quickly.'

'Gosh, it is quick, isn't it? He's just slipped away. That was very peaceful,' he added, still stroking Gus's now flaccid neck and his inert body. However, quick as it was to induce apnoea and render him unconscious, and despite the large dose I had given, Gus's heart kept on beating. He was clinging on to life, despite being totally unconscious and slipping away under the effects of my drug. Under normal circumstances this isn't a problem; as the barbiturate courses round the veins, the heart eventually slows and then stops. In horses and sheep in particular, it can take many minutes before this happens. Sometimes vets give a second dose, just to be safe. Which reminds me . . .

Not long after we had graduated, a friend of mine was called to euthanise a pony. He gave dose after dose, but the pony just stood there in front of him, stubbornly refusing to die. As his and the owner's stress levels rose higher and higher, and as the young vet began to panic that he didn't have sufficient barbiturate left in his vehicle, it finally became clear that the catheter he had placed in the pony's neck was not actually residing within the vein and that the two bottles of barbiturate he had administered had therefore seeped harmlessly into the connective tissues under the skin. There was no wonder the pony was still standing.

Eventually, the job was done, with a peaceful end, lots of tears and even a hug. Notwithstanding, that particular vet now works in the veterinary pharmaceutical industry, far away from the possibility of any clinical calamities. But back to Gus . . .

While on this occasion I knew that my catheter was safely in Gus's vein, more time was not a luxury we had, as Dave's walkie-talkie had twittered into action with a group of trekkers returning to the farm and placing their orders for drinks. They'd be back any minute, chatting excitedly about their trekking experience, which, I can confirm, is a great day out. It would certainly spoil their llama experience if they witnessed the demise of an old favourite in the barn where they'd soon be drinking tea.

'Quick!' exclaimed Dave. 'The trekkers are coming. We can't let them see us putting down Gus!' There was no time to move him to another part of the farm. 'Let's cover him up with straw. Nobody will see him.'

So, as Gus slipped away to wherever llamas go next, snug under a thick blanket of straw, another camelid catastrophe drew to a close. While they are not naturally accident-prone, these fascinating creatures, with their innate curiosity, do have a knack of causing a drama. Which brings us back to where this chapter started – Cinderella.

I arrived at Jackie's, where she was ready and waiting with the stricken alpaca. Within a few moments, I'd worked out why she was struggling, and I didn't know whether to laugh or cry. This time Cinderella was suffering from another equally bad dystocia, which was preventing the normal birth process developing normally – she had a uterine torsion. This is a condition where the cria-containing uterus is twisted through one hundred and eighty degrees, obliterating the opening of the birth canal. Imagine twisting the packaging at the top of a packet of biscuits to stop them going soft. I closed my eyes as I felt internally to get a sense of the spiralling effect as the vaginal wall came to a dead end. Uterine torsion is a fairly common condition in cattle and a skilful vet can sometimes untwist the uterus, but it's usually very hard. In sheep, it is less common and untwisting is impossible because of the position of the twist, so a Caesarean section is always required. I decided that this was going to be the best option for Cinderella.

This was only the second uterine torsion I'd experienced in an alpaca, but out of a total of only about fifteen deliveries that I'd performed on this species it represented an interestingly high proportion. I explained everything to Jackie and even got her to feel inside, so she'd learn what it felt like and be in a better position for next time.

'Cinderella, you love to give me challenges, don't you?' I said as we made preparations for the Caesarean section. It sounds daunting, but the surgical process is broadly the same as it is in a cow or sheep. In some ways, it's actually easier. The work is not heavy like a calving and, while the risk of a kick is the same, the consequences are not likely to leave the vet with a broken limb, just a focal bruise. And alpacas are much more inquisitive and engaged with their human companions than are ruminants. A sheep will lie, dazed and confused, on a straw bale as the vet does their thing, and will not even show a flicker of surprise when she sees her new lambs, delivered by flank incision rather than by the usual route. 'My goodness, where did those appear from?' is not a sentiment that seems to register in a sheep's small brain. I once performed a cow Caesarean and, while I sutured up the hole through which I'd just delivered an oversized calf, the farmer watched in amazement as the patient happily chewed her cud, in her own contented bovine world, blissfully oblivious to what had just happened.

'Look at that,' the old farmer marvelled. 'She's chewing her cud and all the time you're sewing her insides back together! That's a happy cow! I can't believe it. She's not at all bothered!'

Alpacas, on the other hand, with their huge, dark eyes taking everything in, were always interested in what was going on around them and constantly alert to unusual happenings. As I made my first incision, Cinderella, with eyes like Betty Boop, turned her head, cocked to one side with curiosity, to watch my every move. This was disconcerting at first. I'd never had my surgical work inspected by the patient before, and certainly not while the surgery was actually progressing. With her long and elegantly extended neck arching round to her left flank, she had a superb view of all the action. I felt like asking her to look the other way, for fear of both attracting unnecessary criticism and inducing panic. 'WHAT the HECK are you doing to my insides?' she might have thought. But there was neither. Cinderella watched and blinked as if unable to believe her wide eyes, making the occasional squeak of approval. The whole experience was surreal.

I was soon inside and rummaging for the uterus. It was easy to find. Usually the next step is to make an incision through the uterus over the baby's hock. The hock is easy to hold onto, and making the incision over it means the hole is positioned in the right place to make extraction simple. But those long legs necessitated a pause for thought again. I had to adapt my usual technique or else the hole in the uterus would have been ridiculously large. It was only a minor adjustment and I was soon pulling out the cria. The whole alpaca unravelled to an extended length of about a metre and a half. Fearing whiplash, I carefully caught her head like you do with human babies and, with outstretched arms, lowered the baby onto the straw. Within seconds, the new born cria, quickly christened Julia, lifted her head and wobbled it from side to side. Just like the last baby I'd delivered for Cinderella, she also looked like E.T., but all newborn cria do, so it wasn't a surprise. It had been a truly remarkable process in which to be involved, but there was no time to marvel at nature, and how I had given it a helping hand, because I needed to get on. I had some holes to sew up . . .

8. All Creatures

There's a line in one of the Herriot stories which says: 'if you decide to become a veterinary surgeon you will never grow rich, but you will have a life of endless interest and variety.'

And it is that endless interest and variety in the world of veterinary medicine that captivates not just those of us who are amongst it, but also those who love to read about it, or watch it on TV.

Not a day goes by without a new challenge – a complicated condition that causes the vet to scratch their head, an exotic animal that requires serious extrapolation from first principles (and sometimes a quick trawl of the internet) or an owner with a quirky pet and an unusual request. The interaction of a human with an animal is a fascinating one, and one that exposes the true nature of a person more than anything else. The veterinary surgeon is inextricably involved with these entwined emotions.

Another prominent veterinary surgeon, Peter Rossdale, one of the pioneers of modern veterinary practice and the founder of the most renowned equine veterinary practice in the world – and also an author – has recently become a friend. We often chat, about writing books, about veterinary medicine and about the world in general. In a recent email, he pondered the purpose of writing, and more specifically the purpose of a veterinary surgeon writing. He concluded:

> The motive of a writer for recording his thoughts is unclear, even to the writer. It is not that his thoughts may live after him, but rather that thoughts are transitory and, largely, ephemeral. The discipline of placing them on paper is one to be enjoyed for its own sake. Even if no one reads his text that objective, at least, will have been achieved.

I agree with Peter Rossdale's sentiment. A veterinary life is so full of fascinating stories – both human and animal – it seems a shame not to write them down before they are swallowed up by the passing of time. This was probably the reason that Alf Wight committed his tales to paper, using the typewriter that still resides in the old surgery in Kirkgate, Thirsk, rather than it being a clever plan to pay off his mortgage more swiftly than by TB testing cows.

The characters in these books are not wizards or sorcerers, dragons or elves, but ferrets and foals, cats and cows. The land is not a mystical place with enchanted forests and trees that come to life. In many cases, it seems, their stories are set in rural Yorkshire. For me it is every bit as magical. And so is the endless variety of species we treat.

Boris, Luna, Babs and Betty

'Do you think we could look after a rabbit for a few days?' Anne asked, seizing a moment when she sensed I was in a good mood.

I looked up and raised my eyebrows, and the rest of the story unfolded. I suspected this would be as much of a fait accompli as it had been when the first rabbit arrived chez Norton.

'There's this stray rabbit at the practice,' she explained.

Anne worked part-time in two different practices. One was in Boroughbridge, where I worked too – a quaint North Yorkshire town, nestling in a small backwater of tranquil utopia on the edge of the River Ure. Once upon a time, it was hustling and bustling with stagecoach traffic, a stopping-off place exactly halfway between London and Edinburgh and situated at a strategic crossing point on the river. Those days are long past but that history gives the town its endearing charm. Anne's other job was in a practice in Yarm, which had been just as crucial a town in times gone by, as the major port on the River Tees. Yarm retains some charm, but it is not quite the rural idyll of

Boroughbridge, situated as it is on the outskirts of the large industrial area of Teesside. Not that any of this is relevant to the rabbit, of course, but it explained why Anne had met the rabbit and I had not.

'Someone found him in their garden and brought him in,' she went on. 'He has a microchip, but the telephone number doesn't work. He's obviously been someone's pet and has either been abandoned or he's escaped, and he's at the practice, sitting in a kennel. I wondered if I could bring him home to stay with us for a couple of weeks, just until we've traced his owners? It's got to be better for him to be in our garden, eating grass and breathing fresh air, rather than shut in at the surgery, surrounded by dogs and cats.'

It was a persuasive argument and I could hardly argue, although much as I love rabbits and get a great deal of pleasure watching their rabbit habits, I was not sure we needed another one. That said, Luna, our existing rabbit, was lonely. Her companion had recently died (causing enormous upset to Archie, our youngest son, along with great disappointment that even two vets could not cure everything). And we had a spare hutch. The rabbits could live adjacent to one another, although not in close proximity in case they didn't get on or in case the newcomer passed on any germs.

The next day when I arrived home from work, there was much excitement in the garden. Luna had a friend, albeit a temporary one, and we had another rabbit. Luna is a young, perky and pert female rabbit, white with a few brown spots, and upright and alert ears. She spends her days in a large, outdoor run with various separate houses and a long, curvy tube so she can explore and eat grass. We move the run tube every couple of days so she has plentiful fresh grass. On a weekend, we let her out to roam where she pleases around the garden. She often plays with Emmy, our Jack Russell, who (unusually for this type of dog) is her best friend. It's a good life.

The new rabbit was also white but much larger, fluffy and slightly fat, and lop-eared. He had a gormless expression, partly because of his floppy features, but also because he was actually gormless. He had obviously never encountered grass before. He ate rabbit food voraciously but, when presented with a pen full of grass, had not a clue what to do. He just sat, looking confused. Similarly baffling to him were hay, twigs from the apple tree and mint, basil and rocket from the vegetable patch – all things that most rabbits would love to eat. The kids quickly dubbed him Boris, after the recently elected mop-head leader of the Conservative Party.

We watched with interest to see how the two rabbits would react to one another. Boris had testicles and clearly had every intention of making use of them. Even though Luna was spayed (by me, early in her life, to prevent unnecessary diseases), Boris was not deterred from attempting to mate. Even from the next-door hutch, separated by two layers of mesh, his intentions were clear. On top of this, and underneath his harmless exterior, he had rather belligerent tendencies, stomping and kicking in objection when he could not get what he wanted.

As the days passed in Thirsk, Luna was getting more excited about the prospect of having a friend and Boris was getting more sexually frustrated. Meanwhile, back in Yarm, no owner had been forthcoming. It looked as if Boris would be staying.

'We should castrate him,' suggested Anne, knowing that this would temper his temper and be crucial for a stable and happy life, wherever that might be.

'Okay, that makes sense,' I agreed, adding, 'You can do him this time.' This was because:

A) Boris was Anne's idea.

B) I had operated on all our other pets: first Paddy the
Border Terrier was castrated; then Emmy our Jack
Russell was spayed and stitched up after an attack by her
nemesis Maisie; then Luna, the most challenging, was
spayed. Archie had been particularly anxious about this,
given rabbits' less than perfect reaction to anaesthesia.

It was definitely Anne's turn to do the deed and we made arrangements to castrate Boris the following week at the Boroughbridge surgery. I gave him his injection of anaesthetic and presently he was fast asleep in his kennel. I carefully lifted the slumbering lop into theatre, where Anne was ready to do the operation. My only involvement was to clip the hair off his testicles. While this sounds like an easy job, the skin of a rabbit's scrotum is wafer-thin and easily torn or scarified; but every trace of fluffy scrotal hair needs to be taken off, or else fluff will contaminate the wound. Soon, hairless, smooth and clean, Boris's balls were ready to be incised. As he lay on his back his ears gave the impossible appearance of being pricked up to attention. I took a photo because it was comical. I was enjoying being a surgical spectator, and watched Anne do her precise work with scalpel and scissors. It was slick and efficient, although I couldn't help but offer comments about her surgical style, which was on reflection probably not very helpful. It was relaxing to watch rather than do, for a change.

It was soon done and before long Boris was sitting up with his head in a pile of tasty greenery, none of which he knew was food for a rabbit. Confused as usual, he used the pile of herbage as a comfy and fragrant pillow.

Back home, we kept him separate from Luna for a few weeks, to give his hormones time to subside. We put the two runs close to one another though, so the two could see and smell each other. Luna was pleased to see him back and Anne and I, as well as the kids, really hoped he'd stay. The next hurdle was how the pair would get on when they were introduced without a wire netting barrier . . .

While watching the castration of your new rabbit, under the charge of your wife, might have been relaxing, the feeling of responsibility is altogether more considerable when there is a whole classroom full of small children who are besotted by the pet upon whom you are about to operate. This was the case with Babs, a guinea pig who, along with her sister, Betty, belonged to the local primary school. Concern had developed that Babs' abdomen was expanding. A trip to the vets was required, and the teacher came in with both guinea pigs for a check-up and a comparison.

Sure enough, Babs was almost twice as round as her sister, so something was clearly wrong. I decided to perform an ultrasound scan, which confirmed the presence of a huge cystic structure on Babs' right ovary. I relayed the diagnosis to the headmistress and outlined the various options for treatment. I could inject a drug to stimulate the follicle to ovulate, which might effect a cure. I could drain the cyst using a long needle attached to a large syringe, which would again offer a temporary improvement. The best solution however, albeit more risky, would be to spay Babs, removing both ovaries as well as the uterus. This would be a permanent cure, but there was a significant risk involved in both the anaesthetic and the surgery. To put this into context, the chance of an adverse anaesthetic event in a dog is about one in two thousand. In a guinea pig this rises to about one in thirty, so while it is far from dangerous it is markedly more risky to give a general anaesthetic to a guinea pig than to a dog. The head teacher decided that the best thing to do would be to discuss

Babs' treatment with her staff and also the pupils – an excellent exercise in group discussion, even for six-year-olds.

The following day, I received confirmation that the staff and pupils had decided that we should go ahead with surgery. I took a deep breath and felt my pulse quicken; there was an awful lot at stake. It wasn't just the one-in-thirty statistic, it was the knowledge that if things didn't go to plan, the whole school would be upset.

The teacher and a class representative came in with Babs and Betty came too. The two guinea pigs lived together and we decided that having a bestie – if not to say a beastie – there to offer support pre- and post-op would be a good thing.

Betty enjoyed the pre-anaesthetic tasty food, even though she wasn't having an anaesthetic! Babs was soon whisked away from her friend and asleep on the table, where I shaved her huge, distended tummy. I was nervous, and so was my nurse, as I made the first cut. Spaying a guinea pig is a high-pressure piece of surgery and not at all routine. Lots can go wrong. Luckily, during surgery like this I am able to put the emotional attachment of the owners at home or, in this case the children at school, to the back of my mind, so I can focus fully on the task in hand.

Once I had to remove the cancerous eye of an elderly cat called Gizmo, in full knowledge that his owners had dropped him off at the surgery and then gone to the local church to pray for a happy outcome while I excised the eyeball. Again, I had to switch off from the owner's anxiety as best I could. Whether it was good luck, precise surgery or divine intervention, Gizmo made a complete recovery. I hoped Babs would do the same, because I felt a similar weight of responsibility today.

As soon as I cut through the abdominal wall, the huge, cystic structures on the guinea pig's ovaries burst out of the incision. They were impossible to miss, tight like a water balloon and ready to burst. I had to be delicate, precise and swift. The quicker

I had the ovaries out and ligated and the rest of the uterus removed, the better her chances would be. As was usual when an exciting piece of surgery was occurring, I had a camera pointing at my scalpel and me. There was no need to hype up the tension and the persistent questions from the producer-director, eager for soundbites about how serious the problem was, did not help. At one point, I had to ask him to be quiet and stop asking questions. Babs and her ovaries demanded my full concentration. Finally, everything was out and I sutured the gaping hole in her abdomen back together as quickly and neatly as I could. Babs had made it this far.

Before long, the little guinea pig was snuffling and squeaking and looking around. I had two more important jobs to do. The first was to return her to her best friend Betty and the second was to make the all-important phone call to the school to tell them the good news. It was a brief conversation, curtailed by a teacher trying to avoid welling up with tears of relief – although she blamed it on wanting to go and tell the class as soon as possible.

Some weeks later, I was invited to the primary school to carry out a final post-operative check on the patient. I arranged it for an afternoon, just before going-home time, and I sensed the school was excited about the prospect of a visit from a vet. School visits are great and I wish I had time to do more of them. All children love animals and to meet a real life 'animal doctor', complete with stethoscope, offers a brilliant insight into a working life. Today the class was even more excited because the animal doctor in question had saved one of their beloved guinea pigs. I was ushered into the class, which fell silent immediately. I said hello, introduced myself and sat on an unfeasibly small sofa. Ceremoniously, Betty and Babs were brought in, each pig sitting regally on a velvet cushion carried by a capable six-year-old (with teachers close behind, in case of accident or trip). Neither Babs nor Betty looked remotely out of place on their cushions. If they could have raised a forelimb to offer a royal wave, then I would not have been very surprised. I smiled widely, but tried not to laugh. The two guinea pig monitors sat beside me on the small sofa and stroked their pigs. Next, I was presented with a large card made by the children, saying *Thank you Julian*, with an orange-coloured guinea pig on the front. Finally, slices of cake were distributed to everyone apart from the animals. I talked a bit about looking after guinea pigs and explained about the problem from which Babs had suffered, but the six-year-olds didn't seem very interested in cystic ovaries. I asked some questions but, as is often the case when addressing groups of young children, they replied with a string of fairly arbitrary statements rather than answers to what I'd asked.

'I've got a cat.'

'My rabbit died.'

'My dog fell in the pond.'

'I had a mouse but it died.'

The most successful part of my school trip, apart from the cake, was offering the kids a chance to listen with my stethoscope. Babs and Betty were willing volunteers – up to a point, after that it was easier to let the children listen to their own hearts. One by one, when the instrument allowed them to hear their own heartbeat, their eyes would open wide with amazement. All too quickly, the bell rang and everyone rushed out, looking for their parents to take them home. I hoped they'd had an interesting afternoon. I think they did. They were certainly pleased that their favourite guinea pig was better, although I don't think any of them fully appreciated how tense it had been just three weeks earlier.

* * *

Meanwhile in our garden, another pair of patients had been sitting it out, watching each other from separate pens, as Boris's hormone levels subsided. Quite quickly he had stopped stomping his feet, but would he become a suitable companion for Luna? As week three approached for them, it was time to introduce the rabbits in person. We'd been observing their behaviour across the wire netting and they both seemed happy, but the proof of the pudding was whether they'd happily cohabit. With tasty grass and a pile of hay as distraction, we lifted Bulky Boris into Luna's pen and stood back. There was some sniffing, but also obvious mutual respect, and no antisocial behaviour at all. It was the start of a very happy relationship.

Within weeks the two rabbits were inseparable and Boris was flourishing. Now, his dietary repertoire is unimpeachably healthy and his palate is sophisticated. Yes, he still likes his rabbit pellets but, between hopping around the lawn and surveying the scenery from the top of the hutch, he's eating his way through most of the herbaceous plants in our garden. Boris has certainly landed on his feet!

Ferrets

I've loved ferrets all my life. My first pet was a ferret. I called him Fangface, and I was eleven years old when I took custody and care of this feisty little creature.

One Saturday afternoon there was a ring of the doorbell, which usually meant one of my mates was calling to see if I was 'lekking' out. Lekking was the Castleford word for playing. It must have been a word derived from our Viking ancestors, because there is a Scandinavian word, 'leka', that means play. Incidentally, this is also where the term *fartlek* comes from – it means 'speed play' in Swedish and is used to describe a type of interval training used in athletics, a method with which I became very familiar in my teenage years. But in 1980s Castleford, lekking out usually involved a bike or a football, or sometimes nothing other than a sense of adventure.

Anyway, this particular afternoon it was my friend Mark at the door, but he did not have his usual BMX – a Raleigh Burner – and he wasn't there to lek. He was standing on the doorstep with a small wooden box in his hands.

'I've brought you this,' he said, thrusting it forward like children on doorsteps do when they have things to give.

'Someone found it up in the allotments and I know you've been wanting one for ages, so I thought you should have it. If you want it, like.'

Mark was right – I had wanted a ferret for ages, although I hadn't been actively seeking one. As a small boy, I don't think I really knew where one would get a ferret. I had, however, spent many months working out what I would need to keep a ferret, should one miraculously appear, and I had embarked on a construction project. I had found (at the nearby tip) an old wooden cabinet, upright and sturdy, complete with about four sliding drawers. I reckoned the most cost-effective way (in fact, it was free) of acquiring a ferret house was to convert this chest of drawers. I remember planning, sawing, nailing and adapting it into something suitable for the king of ferrets. I remember it taking ages, and I remember it being painstaking because I was eleven and not experienced or adept with hammers and saws. To be honest, even as an adult I am still not adept with hammers and saws.

So that's where Fangface lived – in a converted chest of drawers. I've tried to find photos of Fangface and his house, but to no avail. All I have to rely on is memories. One thing that did bring him back to reality was a letter found by my dad, dated 13 March 1983. At this time, I was ten and had, bizarrely, written a letter to my sister, Kate, who was away on a school trip to Hornsea. I must have thought she would like a letter to stave off the pangs of homesickness. I think the letter says a lot about me, even at that young age.

It went like this:

To Kate,

I went to a race on Saturday with Dad and Sebastian Coe broke a record. I got some autographs and saw Ron Pickering and Geoff Capes. On Sunday, we went to see Castleford play Hunslet at Rugby League and Castleford won.

I have nearly finished making the ferret hutch. I have painted it, put a new floor in and put something to separate the run and sleeping compartment.

From Julian x

P.S. Sorry about my handwriting.

I have reread this letter recently and I don't think the handwriting was that bad. It is actually much better than my present-day handwriting, and the letter is a record of the time in my life when ferrets (and consequently animals in general) started to become really important to me.

In fact, at this time, ferrets filled much of my life. Another friend, Jason, who lived just five houses up the street, kept several of these creatures, too. I would visit him most days during the sunny summer holidays, talk ferrets, learn about feeding and husbandry, lift them out of their pens and learn how to handle them, between shooting tin cans with Jason's air rifle and defying death on our BMXs. They were happy times, before mobile phones and home computers, when the only concern we had was whether we'd be home in time for tea. I learnt a lot about friendships, a bit about air rifles, a bit about doing jumps on BMXs and a lot about ferrets.

Sadly, Fangface's enjoyment of my home-made hutch was relatively short-lived. Jason borrowed him one day to go out en masse with his ferrets, and he never returned. He escaped, running off to look for adventure and excitement no doubt. I was a bit sad, but a pet ferret that lived in an adapted wooden filing cabinet, with a boy about to start grammar school, was never going to live a life that would satisfy a ferret's wanderlust. Fangface would be having his own adventures somewhere in the rabbit holes of West Yorkshire, I thought, and he would be happy. He'd brought much happiness during our short relationship and, looking back, he probably cemented a life working with animals. Thank you Fangface!

Thirty-five years on and at the practice in Boroughbridge, I was treating a lot of ferrets. Many of them belonged to Mrs Turner, ferret fan, ferret rescuer and ferret rehomer. She would come over from Wharfedale almost every week to have her charges checked, spayed, medicated or examined. It was a long and time-consuming journey, but she was happy to make it as she had previously had great difficulty finding a vet with an enthusiasm for this creature, let alone any specific knowledge. Their sharp teeth and quicksilver reflexes put off many veterinary surgeons. But there are many animals with both these attributes that we still look after, so I find this a rather lame excuse. I suspect the smell, lingering, persistent and chemically toxic, might deter some. Ferrets are curious and amazing creatures and a pleasure to treat, but undeniably often very smelly. A case of owner beware.

The smelliest, and also the most fiddly of ferret jobs for a vet, is to perform a vasectomy. It requires careful handling of the testicles and surrounding area to identify the tiny duct called the vas deferens, and then to ligate and transect it. It sounds an odd thing to do for a male ferret – why not just castrate him – but it can be very helpful for the health of the females. Female ferrets, or jills, come into season (or oestrus) in the spring and (like alpacas) are induced ovulators, remaining in season over the summer until they are mated. This maximises their chances of becoming pregnant and therefore has an evolutionary advantage. But it has a disadvantage too. During oestrus, the high levels of oestrogenic hormones have a suppressive effect on the female's bone marrow. If a female ferret is not mated, this suppression can lead to a profound anaemia that can be fatal. The answer is either to prevent them coming into season (by using injections of another hormone or by spaying), or to ensure that they are mated. But without intervention, the latter would result in a population explosion in the ferret world. Using a vasectomised male (a hoblet), that is sexually active but incapable of making a female pregnant, is an excellent solution.

So, when dealing with ferrets a vet needs to be cautious. The phrase 'I would like my hob to be *done*' needs much discussion and clarification with the owner to determine whether they intend their ferret to be castrated – in which case his mating days are done, but he smells much sweeter – or vasectomised, in which case he can continue to mate for the rest of his days, safe in the knowledge that he is actually saving the lives of his harem while doing so.

I have done the procedure many times and there are pitfalls galore. The operation needs to be done in spring, when the testicles expand and the vas deferens swells. In winter, in much the same way as they do for a cyclist out on the hills on a cold, damp day, the gonads shrivel and the procedure is impossible as the structures are too small to see, let alone remove.

I can still recall and still feel the horror of my first attempt to perform a vasectomy on a ferret. I was unaware of the seasonal imperative and it was a snowy day in January. All I could find were tiny strands of tissue; they were indistinct in every way, but I felt certain the correct strands had been removed and so carefully added them to a pot of formalin. This was to preserve them for later, in case of litigation in the face of an unplanned pregnancy. It is something we always do when vasectomising rams, where a mistake can have disastrous consequences if the wrong father sires a whole crop of lambs.

Several months later an irate and red-faced ferret owner stomped into the waiting room, with a mother and father ferret and a box of tiny baby ferrets. I'd clearly removed the wrong bits; there was no need for histological analysis of the strands to confirm my error. It was very uncomfortable and all I could do was apologise. It was not a mistake I made again. I'd learnt another lesson and added it to experience. Again.

My ferret knowledge was called into action again when I arrived back at the surgery one afternoon to start appointments. As I peered out of my consulting room door, I could see a perplexed-and anxious-looking gentleman, sitting at the far end of the waiting room, clutching a plastic bag. No pet, just a plastic bag.

He was first on the list and in big, bold letters next to his name there was a request to see a senior vet. A pet-less client requesting to see the boss usually meant there had been some sort of veterinary mistake (for example, the failure to correctly vasectomise a hob) for which redress was required. Either that, or something very unusual or complicated.

With some trepidation, I called the tall, elderly and perplexed gentleman into the consulting room, where he placed the plastic bag on the table.

'What seems to be the problem?' was my opening gambit, unsure where this consultation would take me.

'Well, Julian. Thank you for seeing me this afternoon. I have something of a mystery,' the man explained. I relaxed, realising with relief that there was no veterinary error to explain away.

'For the last few months, my dog has been acting very strangely, in the night and during the day. His food has been disappearing from the kitchen, even when he's not been in the room. I was very confused, but I started to realise that there may be an *intruder* coming into my house, upsetting the dog and eating his food.'

I didn't see quite why this was a veterinary problem, but he continued, 'And then I found this on the drive.'

He opened the outer layer of what close up looked like a trio of plastic bags.

'And I think this was the culprit. I found it dead just the other day. The food has stopped disappearing and the dog is more settled. But this is a *mystery animal.* I have absolutely no idea what it is – I've never seen anything like it in my life. I've searched up pictures on the internet but I'm stumped. That's why I brought it to show you. I hoped you'd know what it was – just out of curiosity.'

He unpeeled the final layer of plastic as if displaying lost treasure, and I felt rising excitement at the possibility of inspecting a new type of creature, first discovered in North Yorkshire in 2017. I was already planning my phone conversation with the Natural History Museum or David Attenborough.

Sadly, there was no new, undiscovered species inside the three layers of plastic, just a perfect example of an albino ferret! Not unlike my Fangface in appearance – and also in his lust for an adventurous life – he must have escaped. After a bid for freedom, the poor ferret must have sought temporary refuge with this chap and his Labrador, before meeting with a premature end.

Although slightly deflated, at least the man was pleased to find out the identity of this creature, and the mystery was solved. Maybe he was slightly embarrassed at his obvious and silly mistake – that it was simply a common or garden (or kitchen) ferret.

The Birds

It was only after I'd been practising as a vet for almost twenty years that I realised the importance of birds. Or, being more precise, the importance of the bond that can form between a human being and a bird. I feel remiss not to have spotted this, now obvious, connection sooner.

I began to notice the strength of the bond that forms between an owner and a bird, whether it is a parrot, a hen, a swan or a goose, when I started filming for *The Yorkshire Vet* in April 2015. For the first time, I witnessed owners being asked very direct and personal questions, which demanded answers that probed their emotions. Questions like, 'So what does John mean to you?' In that case, John was a swan. Or, 'How important is it that Henny makes a full recovery?' Henny was (obviously) a hen. One terrible Saturday night, Henny had been mauled by a terrier. She had fled her attacker and it took her owners until Sunday lunchtime to find her. The gaping wounds on her back demanded my attention. The irony of treating a chicken on a Sunday lunchtime, at exactly the same time that I should have been sitting down with my family to tuck into my own, roasted version, was hard to ignore.

The searching questions asked by the various producer-directors, who have filmed my clients and me over the years, have delved more deeply into the thoughts and feelings of worried owners than a clinician ever could. Clinicians focus intently on achieving a diagnosis and effecting a treatment plan, and it is all too easy to overlook the psychological aspects of the human-animal relationship, whether that relationship is between an elderly lady and her cat or a farmer and his prize bull. It quickly became clear to me that there is a particularly strong and deep bond between owners and the birds for which they care. It's not immediately obvious why this should be. Maybe it is because of the way birds imprint on a significant other, focusing all their attention on one being. Chicks do this as an innate response shortly after they leave the egg, fixating on the object upon which they first focus. Of course, this is usually their mother and, as such, imprinting is an evolutionary adaption to keep the chick safe. Herring gull chicks can, apparently, be trained to devote themselves to a yellow lollipop stick with a red blob painted on it, mimicking the pattern on the mother's beak, and I have also heard that jackdaws and magpies can be trained to identify and focus on the faces of terrorists and will squawk and riot if these individuals are spotted in a crowd.

This strong feeling was never so evident than with Dougie, the Amazonian parrot. With his magnificent plumage, as green as all the accoutrements in his owner Margaret's kitchen, he found fame via *The Yorkshire Vet* by virtue of having a broad Yorkshire accent. The friendship between Dougie and Margaret had even trumped Margaret's marriage. I called in to see them one day when passing Margaret's house on a quiet afternoon, and realised that Dougie had not only a devoted love for his owner but a vicious hatred of anyone else. He swore at me as I stood in the hall, and flexed his talons in my general direction. Nobody could get between him and Margaret. But I have told the story of Dougie, his Yorkshire accent and his besotted owner before. So, from parrots to geese.

More recently, an extra appointment on my morning's list caught my attention:

Two geese, injured by dogs

It sounded more interesting than the two dogs with diarrhoea, the Labrador with conjunctivitis and the couple of cats in need of their annual vaccinations. To see one goose was unusual but to see two injured geese together . . . I cleared the waiting room so that the other patients, especially the dogs, did not frighten them.

The birds, a goose and a gander, were soon sitting calmly in the waiting room. One was in a cardboard box, wearing one of those close-fitting outfits that babies wear. The other was in a laundry basket, with a pillowcase over its head. It was quite a sight.

It transpired that a pair of terriers who lived on the owner's farm, employed mainly to control the rat population, had taken a liking to, or rather, had developed a vendetta against, the geese. Most dogs would steer well clear of a couple of belligerent geese, but the pair of Border Terriers had obviously egged one another on. The result was some nasty injuries to both goose and gander. The terriers, on the other hand, were unscathed, although (quite literally) in the doghouse.

I examined the male goose first, carefully removing the pillow-case from his head. He looked like a hostage, being smuggled away from the scene by the goose police. But a pillowcase over the head keeps a bird calm when in unfamiliar surroundings – a car journey to the vets, for example – and it also keeps the snappy beak away from the farmer's and the vet's fingers.

His handsome face showed not a trace of distress as he looked around, checking out things to peck at. There was a large wound on his back, where he had borne the brunt of the terrier attack. The female bird, once I'd removed the babygro, had similar injuries.

There was a lot of bruising, damage to the skin and some tissue necrosis, all of which is common with crushing injuries. Worst of all, fly eggs and little maggots had appeared in the dead and damaged tissue. It took a painstaking half an hour to rid Mr and Mrs Goose of all the maggots I could find. It is a grim, but strangely satisfying job and all vets have their favoured technique. Mine is to use forceps to get the obvious ones. I then apply blue spray to the wound. When squirted vigorously, the horrible grubs soon panic and emerge to the surface, desperate for air, and I can get to work with my forceps again.

The wounds were soon clean, and after a couple of injections both goose and gander had a much more favourable prognosis. I helped carry them to the car. The female sat comfortable and safe in her box, carried by her owner. She could not see her surroundings, but the gander – now pillowcase-less – in his lidless laundry basket, which I was carrying, knew exactly where he was. He made a bid for freedom, jumping and flapping at the same time. Luckily, I managed to grab him, but as the consequences of a successful escape ran through my mind, some words from a Mr Men book I used to read to my kids popped into my head. *There's a goose, loose in the lane!* Thankfully, a loose goose disaster had been averted.

Of course, some bird owners are less emotionally attached. Perky the pigeon had been with us for a couple of days and had already made himself comfortable in a quiet corner of the kennels. Perky wasn't his real name, but his only other form of identification was the number on the ring on his leg. It didn't seem very nice to refer to this racing pigeon simply by his number, so we called him Perky. But while Perky *was* fairly perky, he was not really very good at racing. He had been found by a passer-by, sitting on a village green just outside Boroughbridge. Many tourists had been doing a similar thing during the warm summer months, some having travelled long distances to get here. We did not know where Perky's journey had started, but it must have been a long way away, because he was tired, hungry and dehydrated when he was brought into the surgery.

The lost pigeon was just one of the waifs and strays under our care at the time. At the opposite end of the kennels was a hedgehog who had been found, equally bewildered and in a place where he shouldn't have been, out and about during the daytime. Just like a racing pigeon sitting on the village green, a hedgehog out in the daytime is clearly in trouble, and it was right that he had been brought in for veterinary attention. The hedgehog had been given the name Horace, after the 1980s computer-game character Hungry Horace, who crossed roads trying to avoid the traffic and find things to eat. Horace the hedgehog had narrowly avoided a similar fate to his computer-game namesake, and when we checked him over, the spiky character's problems were very evident. Horace was covered in ticks, each one the size and shape of a piece of sweetcorn, full of the little hedgehog's blood, which the nasty parasites had been sucking to engorge themselves before detaching and laying lots of eggs. The result was severe anaemia for Horace. Every tick needed painstakingly to be removed. It had been another job for the forceps but, once he was tick-free, we were confident that with a bit of rest, recuperation and cat food he would make a full recovery.

Perky the pigeon was also gaining strength. He had been eating and drinking well and looked altogether healthier. We'd even managed to find a telephone number for his owner via the identification number on his leg ring.

Sally, one of the nurses, called the owner to pass on the good news that we had found his pigeon and find out what he wanted us to do with him. I guessed the owner might not be as excited as we hoped, because a pigeon that didn't return home was surely not a very good homing pigeon. There was a possibility that he wouldn't want him back at all.

After several abortive attempts, Sally eventually managed to make contact. To our relief, Perky's owner, who was based in Derbyshire, was pleased his missing pigeon had been found and delighted that it had regained strength after a period of rest.

So, asked Sally, what should we do with Perky?

She was surprised at the answer: 'Just chuck it up, duck!'

After morning ops had been finished, we took Perky the pigeon outside and found a space clear of roads and traffic. He'd had a good drink and some breakfast, so we all held our breath and, as instructed, 'chucked it up'. Mercifully, well rested and well fed, like all the horses that had stopped overnight in Boroughbridge centuries ago, Perky made his way south. I hoped his owner would be pleased to have him back!

Squeaky the swan was a bird who was right up there when it came to avian-human interdependence.

Jackie had a couple of swans who were totally in love with each other. Squeaky and John, both black swans, were inseparable, just like Odette and Siegfried in the famous ballet *Swan Lake*.

But Jackie came a very close third in the relationship.

Jackie's husband was a retired engineer with a passion for digging holes to facilitate drainage solutions. On each of the several occasions I'd visited their house – either to check on swans, vaccinate a dog or examine a lame pony – he had been beavering away on his mini-digger, making drainage ditches and interconnecting ponds and larger lakes. It was in (or on) one of these lakes that Squeaky and John lived, along with a selection of less affectionate waterfowl.

One day Squeaky was spotted looking limp and weak on a small island in the middle of their lake. Jackie had gone out in a little rowing boat to investigate, and could see that her left wing was badly damaged. An amphibious rescue was undertaken, followed by a trip to the vets.

Jackie arrived carrying a large cardboard box under her arm, wrapped up like a rustic Christmas present, with string tied in a bow. I pulled on one end of the string to untie it and a sock appeared out of the box. The sock was animated, just like the one that contained a mouse in the children's story of Kipper and his toy box. (Some of you will know what this means. If you don't, I urge you to look up the story. It's very funny.) Inside the sock was Squeaky's head, which fitted perfectly. The purpose of the sock, a bit like the goose's pillowcase, was to keep the swan calm and relaxed on the journey and to allow easy examination, free from unwanted pecking. I didn't mind the pecking, though, and removed the sock so Squeaky could see me. Like many an avian fan, I found myself anthropomorphising my patient and introduced myself before starting to examine the wing. Both it and the wound around its base were irreparable. It would need to be amputated.

Now, amputating the wing of a bird is not something to be taken lightly. In fact, it is positively the last resort, as it renders flight totally impossible. Some amputations are well tolerated. A waterbird with just one foot, for example, could still paddle itself about (at least in a circular pattern). A four-legged animal with one limb removed can hop along quite comfortably and generally will cope incredibly well. But removing a wing is another thing altogether. However, luckily for Squeaky, there was a good chance she could manage without the appendage. She barely flew anywhere. Most of the time her wings were folded across her back, ornamentally arched as she swam with grace, following John. The defunct wing would not be missed. I arranged to see Squeaky the following day for the surgery.

Again, she arrived at the practice with her head in a sock,

quiet and comfortable. This time, I left the sock in place and took her to theatre and applied the gas mask to her sock, toe-end first. The camera crew, consisting of Laura with her camera and Rory capturing sound on his fluffy boom microphone, were there too. Everything was going smoothly, even though this was the first time I had removed a swan's wing (did I *really* need to seek consent from the Queen?).

I'd made the first incisions and Laura zoomed in for a close-up of the wing coming off. Just at this very point, I caught a large artery – it must have been the left subclavian, although its name was the last thing on my mind at this stage – and blood began to spurt rhythmically and persistently, curving in a perfect arc over my surgical kit right onto the very expensive camera lens and down the front of Laura's equally expensive designer white linen top.

'Stop! Stop!' cried Laura, laughing, more concerned about whether her footage would be obscured by streaks of Squeaky's crimson blood than about her expensive top.

I laughed too, but I had more pressing matters than the quality of Laura's images. I managed to clamp the pumping vessel with a pair of artery forceps and order was restored.

Squeaky made a remarkable recovery and, after a suitable period housed in isolation from John and away from the murky waters of the pond, she was ready for a reunion with both. I went to watch, accompanied by Laura and her camera. The two lovebirds reconnected immediately, entwining their long necks. They walked towards their pond and slid in together in perfect unison. It felt as if two lives had been saved, rather than just Squeaky's. I paused on the side of the pond. Was I becoming just a little bit sentimental when it came to treating birds? I smiled to myself and tossed bits of food to them across the water. Maybe I was, but I didn't mind.

We're All Going to the Zoo Tomorrow

It was one of my first days at middle school and the assignment for the afternoon was to draw a picture of your favourite animal. For some reason, I can remember this day very well. I can easily bring to mind the pile of plain paper in the centre of an octagonal and short-legged table, and the pots of coloured pencils nearby. That day, I drew a tortoise, which I knew was cheating. A tortoise was most definitely *not* my favourite animal – I'm not sure I had even seen a tortoise in real life, let alone formed a meaningful relationship with one. My cousin used to keep terrapins, which are the amphibious version, but they held little attraction for me. They showed no affection and their life in a small heated tank, full of partly submerged rocks, thermometers and artificial lights, did not seem very meaningful.

What prompted me to draw a tortoise on that particular early day at school were two things. Firstly, I was rubbish at art and found it difficult to make anything look remotely realistic. I knew very well that if I tried to draw a picture of my favourite animal, which was a dog, the poor creature would look like a sausage or a freak. Secondly, I knew drawing a tortoise should be easy because half of its body was a vague semicircle, its head was similar in shape to a sausage (which I could draw quite well) and the legs emerging from under the semicircle were so short as to present no artistic challenge, even to a drawing dunce.

Sadly, my picture did not survive the passage of time and tidy-ups, but I recall my parents being extremely impressed by this piece of work. The biggest effect it had on them was unbridled amusement as I'd made the pragmatic decision to draw something simple and defy the objectives set out by the teacher. Fortunately, it was not a habit I continued and I eventually became a model pupil, albeit one with a pragmatic streak and no artistic ability.

But now, as a veterinary surgeon, I find that I have developed an enthusiasm for tortoises that I would never have expected, although when I see one it always reminds me of my most famous piece of artwork and the mirth of my parents. Tortoises are very interesting animals and, possibly because they live for such a long time (in fact, they are the longest-living of all land animals), they have huge personalities, individually evolved over decades and, from a species point of view, evolved over millennia.

Because of this longevity, it always feels as if there is extra pressure and added responsibility when treating a tortoise. This was particularly so with Toby, a septuagenarian chelonian who had been bequeathed to his new owners in a will. Pam had taken the casual vacancy that was Toby's ownership and, when I met her for the first time before Toby's first hibernation, she was worried.

'Julian, I do feel very *responsible* all of a sudden,' she confessed. 'I don't really know much about tortoises and Toby is older than I am. Not by much, mind.'

On this occasion, I had assumed the role of tortoise expert in the practice. One colleague, who was from Spain, pronounced the name of the animal in the same way as you'd pronounce the colour turquoise, and claimed to know absolutely nothing about the species. Even if she did know about them, if she couldn't even pronounce the word correctly she would have trouble convincing clients.

So, I checked Toby over – as much as his impenetrable shell would allow. I weighed him and measured him to establish the ratio of length to weight, which would tell us if he was of sufficient size to undergo the hibernation process – a process that apparently involved a large sandwich box and a fridge. I confirmed him as weighty enough, and gave a couple of precautionary and boosting injections of vitamins to keep his levels topped up over the cold winter months. I reassured Pam that, counterintuitive as placing a live animal in a box and then packing it away it in the fridge might seem, it was a good thing to do. It allowed perfect temperature control at exactly the correct level to slow Toby's metabolism. If a tortoise hibernates in a cardboard box in a shed, unseasonal shifts in the temperature, whether global warming or just shed-warming, can be confusing and ultimately catastrophic.

Pam left, clutching Toby under her arm, to head to the hardware shop for a suitable overwintering box.

The next time I met Pam was in the spring. She'd spent the long winter evenings reading and learning about tortoises to equip her to be Toby's custodian in the years to come. He had duly emerged from his slumbers, but he was sluggish and stubbornly refusing to eat. This is called 'post-hibernation anorexia' and can be a challenge to treat. Like a teenager on a Saturday morning, it can be difficult to kick-start the tortoise's body into life. Unlike a teenager on a Saturday morning, frequent warm baths can help, and this was the first thing Pam had done to try to stimulate Toby into action. It didn't help. I checked him over to make sure there were no signs of actual ill-health, such as a mouth infection, or a foot injury sustained by being nibbled by mice during the big sleep (admittedly this was unlikely since Toby had been in the fridge, although it can happen if the tortoise has been hibernating in a shed). He seemed very healthy, but he persistently turned his nose up at the smorgasbord of offerings that Pam had been lining up in front of his wrinkled face.

There was nothing for it but to pass a stomach tube and force-feed Toby. This is not a very nice procedure. First, you have to grasp each side of the tortoise's head very firmly behind its jaws and hold on tightly as the patient tries to pull his head in to evade interference. Tortoises have very strong muscles and can powerfully resist a human's finger and thumb, so there is usually a battle of Carthaginian proportions, and it feels as if you are going to pull its head off! Then, you slide the plastic tube down the oesophagus into the stomach, the sensation of which must feel awful for the tortoise. Toby, as predicted, responded with revulsion, especially as he clearly did not like the taste of the homogenised nutrient mixture; it must have tasted as horrible as it looked. I managed to instil about an eggcup full of the life-giving mush, but was left with a big mess and a tortoise in a sulk, steadfastly refusing to stick out head, tail or limbs from under his shell.

I hoped this small aliquot of energy drink would boost his appetite, but if it didn't I would need a plan B.

Two days later, Toby and Pam were back. He hadn't eaten at all and was now, as well as being on hunger strike, refusing to drink. The only hydration he had had was a few teaspoons of warm bathwater, which had been sucked up into his anus and absorbed *per rectum*. This was going to be tricky.

'Leave him with me, Pam,' I said, as I tried to think what plan B might be.

I decided to pay a visit to the local greengrocer's shop in Boroughbridge. This brilliant shop is called Fink (named after its owner, Hugh Fink), and is as much a delicatessen as a fruit and vegetable emporium. I would seek out a picnic fit for a king tortoise. As ever, I was being filmed by my energetic producer-director Laura. Series seven (or was it eight?) of *The Yorkshire Vet* was being made and a shopping trip to find a feast for an anorexic tortoise would tick a lot of boxes. So I went shopping with a camera and tripod following. I even had a shopping list, consisting of all the tasty things I could think of that might tickle Toby's appetite. Beansprouts, blueberries, coriander, pears and parsnips were all on my list and soon my basket was full. But would it work?

Back at the practice, I arranged everything on a plate and offered each delight to Toby in turn. He pulled his head into his shell in disgust at everything. It looked as if my trip had been in vain and I'd have to reach for the stomach tube again. Laura's camerawork, with nifty pull-focuses and colourful backgrounds, would also be wasted if the patient failed to eat any of my shopping. Eventually, I came up with another idea; a way of making the feast even more tasty. I sliced a blueberry in half, exposing the succulent insides. SUCCESS! Toby's ancient jaws opened as if he was about to do a huge yawn, before he tilted his head and gulped it down. Then he ate the second half, with equal enthusiasm. I was almost dancing with delight. I knew he was on the mend. For pudding, he ate half a beansprout. It felt like the beginning of a story about a caterpillar whose appetite became insatiable.

A few weeks later, partly for the purposes of filming an end scene to the Toby story and partly because I genuinely wanted to see how he was progressing, I arranged to call and see Toby and Pam in their garden. By now, spring had well and truly arrived and the lawn was bursting with dandelions, well known to be the favourite food of tortoises. I lay down on the sunny grass with Toby and hand-fed him freshly plucked dandelions, which he devoured with gusto. Both Pam and I felt the weight of responsibility lift from our shoulders. At last, Toby was thriving.

Maybe it was because of my success with Toby, which had been broadcast on telly, or maybe it was just a coincidence, but a few months later there was a message on my phone from a friend who was the producer of another television programme.

'Julian, I was wondering what you were doing next Tuesday. There is a huge tortoise, he's eighty years old – we think, but nobody really knows for sure – and he's bleeding from somewhere. He's a giant tortoise and the zoo vet is planning to anaesthetise him to find out what is going on. We need an expert presenter and we wondered if you'd like to come and help?'

I picked up the message in the middle of afternoon surgery. I had been busy with normal vet stuff – a lamb with a broken leg, a vomiting dog who needed to be put on a drip and an anorexic cat, which was just as complicated to diagnose and treat as an anorexic tortoise.

All these things I could deal with easily, but this, if I agreed to help, would put me out of my comfort zone for at least two reasons:

A I am not a television presenter,
B I am not an expert on giant tortoises.

I had obviously seen plenty of tortoises before, just like Toby, which I had treated simply. I love dealing with them, but it is not a field I know a huge amount about. I have X-rayed them to look for fractured legs, kidney stones or weak bones and I've amputated a digit from a turtle named Spartacus, when it was bitten by his nemesis Hercules. The last time I had attempted to anaesthetise a tortoise I had watched and waited and watched and waited some more as he completely failed to go to sleep. I did not fancy my chances with a giant version, and it would be worse in this new capacity as a presenter, under the scrutiny of yet another camera. It would certainly be more stressful and much more complicated than buying and slicing a few blueberries.

'But of course,' I found myself saying when I returned the call, 'I'd love to help. That sounds a lot of fun. I have a farm visit on Tuesday morning, but I can try to rearrange it. I'm supposed to be on call on Monday night but I can probably do a swap.'

I had lost touch with the concept of a 'comfort zone' over recent years and, once again, I seemed to have agreed to do something ridiculously unconventional.

I managed to swap my night on call and because the warm, dry weather was more conducive to cutting silage than pregnancy testing cows, the farmer actually rearranged my planned farm visit for me. The next thing I knew I was sitting in the passenger seat of a car loaded with cameras, fluffy booms, spare lights and batteries, miscellaneous other equipment, a producer and a director. There was even a selection of safety boots with steel toecaps, which were part of the risk assessment in case the several-hundred-kilogram patient stood on someone's foot. This would be a very different tortoise from any others I had treated!

I used the long car journey to do some research. I typed 'giant tortoises' into my phone and scanned the results. What I read quickly confirmed that I was definitely not an expert. Luckily, there would be a genuine expert on hand, an exotics specialist whose job it was to provide veterinary care for all the animals at the zoo, from lions to lemurs and rhinos to rabbits. She would be in charge and my job was simply to assist, to ask the appropriate questions at key stages of the procedures and then to provide a comparison to normal veterinary work where appropriate.

The following morning, I met the keeper, who introduced me to 'Biggie' and explained his story and his problem. The geriatric giant was older than anyone at the zoo could remember. His presence pre-dated any of the current staff and nobody had recorded his age when he arrived. Conjecture was that, as my friend had said, he was at least eighty years old. Weighing scales confirmed that he weighed over two hundred and fifty kilograms, hence his name, which he shared with the American rap star. I peered into the hothouse where he lived with his friend, Helen, equally slow but slightly smaller. As Biggie trundled around his tropical house, chewing slowly on herbage, he could not have looked less like a rap star if he tried.

In common with his namesake at the end of his life, Biggie was leaking blood from his body, and reddish stains had been spotted on the floor of the house. However, in contrast to his namesake, it wasn't immediately clear to anyone from where this blood was emanating and today's job was to investigate. The suspicion was that it was coming from his phallus. This is the word used for the male genitalia of a tortoise. It is similar to a mammalian penis, but not exactly the same, and the spade-shaped organ protrudes from the cloaca to allow mating to occur. To examine the phallus and its surroundings, first Biggie needed to be placed under general anaesthetic. The optimistic exotic vet (exotic by speciality, not by demeanour) appeared with huge syringes full of super-concentrated drugs, which had been specially reconstituted from powder to make them much stronger than the stuff I'd use in a regular-sized pet. The last time I'd tried to place a tortoise under anaesthetic it had been a complete failure, so I was not especially hopeful that today's exercise would yield any useful results, but we pressed on regardless. The advantage of Biggie was that he had huge veins, which we hoped would make intravenous injection straightforward. His jugular was the size of a human finger so, if the catheter placement went to plan, we could give him his anaesthetic directly into the vein, which would be very much preferable to the intramuscular technique we tend to use in general practice.

I watched as the exotic vet tried and failed to place the catheter. It didn't look easy and the pressure was all on her, especially with a camera pointing at her and me asking questions all the time. There is a phenomenon we call 'second vet syndrome', where the mere presence of another veterinary surgeon nearby renders the primary vet completely useless. Whatever the reason, Biggie didn't receive the intravenous dose we had hoped for and we had to resort to the slower- (much slower) acting intramuscular route.

I left them to it and wandered off to find an ice cream and unpeel my waterproofs, which were unhelpfully only serving to keep water *inside*. I was already melting from the heat of the summer and the tropical temperature inside Biggie and Helen's house, and my trousers were soaked with sweat. I was regretting opting for my wellies and waterproof trousers – useful on a cold farm in Yorkshire but not useful in a tropically heated reptile house. I made another mental note to wear shorts next time I was called to a reptile house. If there was a next time.

Hours later, and after numerous false alarms ('I think he's asleep now') when motionless Biggie would lift his heavy head and amble away the minute we tried to lift him, he was finally unconscious. With a strong person at each corner of his shell, we managed to manhandle him onto a trolley, which was amusingly and inexplicably not called a trolley by anyone there.

Instead, everyone called it (and kept calling it) a 'dilly', even though it was most definitely a trolley. Off camera, I asked one of the keepers why everyone kept calling the trolley a dilly.

'Because that's what it's called,' came the obvious reply. I didn't probe any further.

Finally, sleeping on the trolley or dilly or whatever it was called, Biggie was rolled into theatre.

More hours passed and more anaesthetic was administered and a tube was finally inserted into his ancient lungs to keep him asleep. Meanwhile, enjoying the fact that my veterinary skills were not actually required today, I squatted at the back end of Biggie and asked probing questions about what might happen when his phallus became extruded. I'd never seen a tortoise's phallus before but I didn't have to wait long before another first. It turned out that his phallus was spade-sized as well as shade-shaped! The tortoise was giant by name and most definitely giant by nature. But there was no sign of bleeding and, even after various other tests, no diagnosis had been made.

Biggie was wheeled out of theatre on his dilly and back to his hothouse, where everybody watched his recovery from the anaesthetic, which took even longer than its induction. I went for another ice cream – progress was painfully slow and by this time I'd run out of incisive questions. Eventually Biggie opened his eyes and his recovery was complete. After about twelve hours of effort, we'd failed to achieve a diagnosis and I'd lost about three kilograms of weight through sweating down my legs and into my wellies. On the journey home, I considered how interesting my day had been and what a very different job the life of a zoo vet was. I'd enjoyed it thoroughly, but give me a consulting room full of standard animals any day, where I'm sure more diagnoses would have been made and more cures effected. If only Biggie's problem had been as simple to fix as a trip to the greengrocers and a handful of berries!

The Last Calving?

The comfort and silence of a peaceful night's sleep was abruptly disturbed by the determined and high-pitched noise of my beeper. I pushed aside the pillow that had been under my knees to keep my rickety lower back stable, rolled sideways and screwed up my eyes to read the message. Would it be a call for advice, with an owner happy to defer an examination of their pet until after daybreak, when everything seems better? Would it be a dog, struggling with seizures in need of urgent assistance? Maybe a cat, out on his nocturnal adventures, who had crossed a road without pausing to look left or right? When a beeper violates your sleep during the dark, small hours, there's a moment of resigned desolation when you realise your job pervades your life. Even when you are deeply asleep, resting and trying to recover from a busy day, recharging before the next day's challenges, there is no place to hide. But I now had an added reason to resent being hauled from my bed. Increasingly, a night's sleep had become critical to allow my dilapidated lumbosacral spine to ease back into some sort of normality. A lifetime of calving cows, lugging heavy dogs onto operating tables and grappling with the sore feet of uncooperative horses had taken its toll on my vertebrae.

I once worked in a practice where the out-of-hours phones were manned by a small company that consisted of two mates who took emergency calls for several different vet practices, all over the country. Occasionally, I'd get the equivalent of a 'wrong number'. *Mr Jones, Valley View Farm, sheep with prolapse* was the message, late one Sunday evening. I didn't recognise the name, and when I called the number on the screen, it became clear that Mr Jones had a hill farm in South Wales and the answering service had bleeped the wrong vet! It was almost worth being disturbed to experience the sense of relief, if not to say actual jubilation, that I got to stay in my warm bed. It was highly unlikely that this would be the case tonight, but I always lived in hope.

This gloom associated with having to get out of bed is usually dispelled by a surge of adrenalin as I realise that I will, quite probably, be saving a life. If it is a ewe to lamb or a cow to calve, two lives might be at stake. There will be a worried farmer, no doubt distressed that he has had to drag a weary vet from his bed, but anxious about his cow. This surge of adrenalin is very helpful and is more powerful than caffeine. Recently though, due to a stream of busy nights on call followed by non-stop days, and because of the ongoing pain in my lower back and legs, which was impossible to ignore, the surge of hormones from my adrenal glands had subsided to more of a trickle. I read the message on the beeper and hoped the trickle would be sufficient to get me through the evening.

Calving. Wilson's. Big calf, lots of legs. Visit please I read, partly digesting the words and partly acting on instinct. It was no wrong number and it was not a job to put off until morning.

I needed to get up and get into action. Lives were at stake. Again.

I pushed aside the pillow that had been in the perfect position under my knees to reduce the nagging pain in my lower back, and rolled sideways. The weather must have changed since I'd gone to bed; heavy rain was lashing at the windows. I could almost feel it. A deep breath, then I fumbled for my clothes, picturing the next few hours of work in my mind.

Like most vets in mixed practice, I'd grown used this. Or, at least, I'd grown accustomed to it. One particularly memorable call occurred during the early days of filming for *The Yorkshire Vet*. It was cold, windy and the middle of the night. I had a camera crew staying nearby in a bed and breakfast, ready to capture the excitement of a night on duty with a Yorkshire vet. Laura and her assistant, Tash, were desperately hoping for some night-time action, though I was hoping for a full night's sleep. I was awoken abruptly, struggled to focus on the message, sighed loudly at the prospect of two or more hours of hard work in the cold and dark, and then called them.

'I have a cow to calve. I can pick you up on the way past. In about ten minutes,' I told Laura, trying to be cheerful, before adding. 'It's at a place called The High Buildings, so it's gonna be cold. Put plenty of clothes on.'

It was cold enough working on farms on a windy December night, but standing relatively stationary, holding a sound boom or a film camera, would be even colder. I'd been chilled to the core on numerous occasions while 'seeing practice' as a vet student, observing and learning but not moving. I didn't want Laura or Tash to freeze. It was bad enough dragging them out of bed.

I drew up outside their digs and watched with increasing amusement as the two TV makers struggled to negotiate their way into my car, each rather like a medieval knight trying to mount a horse.

'I've put on a couple of extra layers, like you said,' explained Laura, plonking herself in the passenger seat before starting to fiddle with her camera, 'Now it's hard to bend my legs. It's actually very difficult to move at all!'

Trees bent and strained under the force of the gale as I negotiated windy lanes and steep hills, but it wasn't long before we arrived at the farm. It was just as well Laura and Tash were so warmly dressed; the wind howled and whistled around the farm buildings, whose name described their position, high up on the top of a hill. On a summer's day this was a beautiful place, but that night it was anything but. The old-fashioned stone barns held little heat at the best of times, but it was even worse than that because the rusty old cattle crush where our patient was restrained was outside the barn, in the full force of the northerly wind. I pondered my plan of attack. Usually, in typical Herriot style, I would remove all the clothes from the top half of my body to gain extra reach into the birth canal and to avoid ruining yet another shirt with bovine bodily fluids. On that night though, as drizzle swirled in eddies around the open fold yard, removing any clothes at all seemed a plainly stupid idea. I donned my waterproof calving top and hoped for the best.

Nobody froze to death and the Caesarean section went to plan, but the calf was not alive. The cloudiness of its eyes told me that it had been dead for some time. There was nothing that could have been done. At least the mum was safe, and the farmer was happy about that, despite the disappointment of not having a strong and healthy calf to show for our night's efforts. Laura and Tash had managed to get some exciting footage to use on *The Yorkshire Vet*, and chatted excitedly as we warmed up in the car on the way home.

But tonight at Mr Wilson's there would be just the farmer and me in the pouring rain and howling gale. I had no camera crew, which was maybe a good thing, because I was tired and sore and definitely not in the mood to smile cheerfully and give a running commentary on the night's events as they unfolded.

I found the farm with some difficulty. I'd been there before, but in the daylight. Everything looked very different after dark and in torrential rain. In the pitch-black farmyard stood a tractor with its lights on and in the beam of those lights was the patient. It was not a great sight. The cow was laid flat out on a mixture of straw and mud, right in the middle of the yard. She had not even made it as far as the calving pen before exhaustion had set in. Pushing and straining is hard work, even for an animal as tough and stoic as a cow.

'Hello,' I said, 'Have we got problems?' It was my standard, non-specific introduction in situations like this one.

'We have,' replied Mr Wilson. 'I'm sorry to call you out on a night like this.'

I was grateful for his apology – he didn't want to be standing in the rain in a muddy farmyard at two o'clock in the morning any more than I did, and his first thought was to acknowledge our mutual inconvenience.

'It's certainly not a very nice night for it!' I added, superfluously.

Mr Wilson briefly described the situation before offering me a bucket of tepid water in which some murky calving ropes were submerged. He'd tried to manipulate the calf himself, without success. I felt inside the mother, although the crossed feet at the cow's vulva and the diameter of said feet led me to conclude that an internal investigation was completely pointless. The calf was clearly huge and I quickly decided I would need to perform an emergency Caesarean. After that, I was more or less on autopilot.

First, I gave the cow an epidural. Eight millilitres of local anaesthetic, injected directly into the fluid surrounding the lower region of the spinal cord, worked wonders to relieve her pain and stop her from straining. It is remarkably simple to effect a good epidural injection in a cow and the effect is instant. Mr Wilson's cow soon had a floppy tail and wobbly legs – not that she could use them, in her stricken position in the mud.

The rest of the job was routine – clipping, cleaning, injecting local to numb the flank, cleaning my arms (although the antiseptic was quickly washed off by the incessant rain), cutting through skin, muscle, peritoneum, finding the uterus, finding the calf's back leg inside the uterus, pulling it up towards the open air, straining, swearing and sweating into the cow's abdomen (despite the cold), pulling, heaving and swearing some more. Then the cow rolled with a lurch in the opposite direction. I let go of the calf's back leg, which was still inside the muscular uterus, as my lower back went into a spasm, sending shooting pains down my legs as far as the underside of my big toes. I bent double, took a few deep breaths to gather my composure and started again, holding the scalpel blade between my teeth so I could use both hands, like some sort of bovine Tarzan but without the vines to swing on. This time I got a better hold and managed to get the calf's leg up. I took the blade from my teeth and made a long, curved incision into the uterus, allowing the calf's foot to burst out into the rainy night. My back screamed again, but this was not the time to stop, and I extended my cut until both feet appeared. I have learnt that it is folly to skimp on the size of the uterine incision; if the opening in the uterus is too small it will only end in problems.

The cow shifted and contracted her abdominal muscles. She was trying to help, trying to push out the enormous calf, but only made matters worse as her rumen bulged out of her side.

I used my forearms to push it back. I felt like one of those musicians playing many different instruments at once, as I tried not to swallow the scalpel blade between my teeth or let it slice the corners of my mouth. Composure was regained as the rumen slid back into the abdomen. I took a moment to deposit the blade back on my surgical kit before I pulled the calf out, backward through the hole I'd recently made in the side of its mother. It was not easy, but compared with the previous half an hour it was plain sailing and, with a slither, the calf landed splat in the mud and immediately started shaking its head and looking around. We were both relieved.

I took a moment or two to stretch before starting the sewing-up process. Another stooped and painful half an hour and I was finally done. Literally done.

I won my customary race to get the side of the cow closed and sealed before the calf was standing. The sooner the abdominal cavity is sealed, the better the chances for the cow. A farmyard is not as hygienic as an operating theatre and, although cows and sheep have an uncanny knack of avoiding infection after such al fresco surgery as tonight's, the sooner everything is closed up the better. Rain only makes it worse, trickling potential infection straight into the cow. The race is only with myself, and in my mind, but it gives me a focus for achieving a slick and efficient conclusion to the op. I nearly always win.

The Simmental calf, with its pretty brown and white face and its already curly coat, was making concerted efforts to stand on its wobbly legs. It would not be long before it was suckling away. We all hoped the cow's maternal instincts would kick in to complete a rewarding night's work.

Rocking back, hands on hips, I exhaled loudly. The griping pain in my lumbar region was not disappearing, nor the shooting pains down my legs. It was a toss-up which was more uncomfortable

– the numbness and strange sensations in my legs or the shooting pains radiating from my buttocks to my big toes. Lower back pain is something pretty much all large animal vets get used to, especially when cold, wet and stooped, pulling an oversized calf out of the side of a cow, reacting and responding to the unpredictable twists and lurches of the mother.

I sprayed the wound with my customary blue spray and gave the necessary injections, before hobbling over to the water trough to clean my arms, torso and wellies. It was the nearest and only water source I could find. It was freezing and unpleasant, but I knew I'd soon be back to the warmth of heated car seats, warming my core and soothing my back.

Unable to soldier on with the pain, I'd recently had an MRI scan. The people in the imaging department at the hospital put the pictures from the scan on a disc for me to take to the surgeon, but they wouldn't let me look at them myself. It wasn't in the hospital rulebook. So, later that evening, I downloaded the appropriate software to allow me to view the images. I'd diagnosed a whole series of serious abnormalities before realising I knew very little about MRI images of a human spine – which was obviously why patients were not supposed to look at them! My diagnosis would have to wait for a few days, until I saw the surgeon.

And that diagnosis was not quite what I'd anticipated. Yes, there was the wear and tear and obliteration of several intervertebral discs that I was expecting, but in addition I had a condition called lumbosacral spondylolisthesis, compounded by a stress fracture to one of my lumbar vertebrae. This was more than just the wear and tear of an active sportsman and overworked vet. This spinal abnormality was the reason my lumbar nerves were being so compressed, and the reason my pain had suddenly escalated to a whole new and horrible level.

My body has held together remarkably well over the years and, compared with many vets, I've had few problems. The worst accidents stick in my mind. A well-aimed kick to my head in my first few weeks as a vet in the north of Scotland left me dazed and mildly concussed but nothing worse. There was a calf that kicked me square in the testicles while I was helping to gather a bunch of cattle for a TB test. It was dramatic but the pain was relatively transient. Various scalpel cuts to the hands have all been simply sewn back together, and I've only contracted a few zoonotic diseases – orf, ringworm, campylobacter, crypto-sporidium and, on several occasions, cases of itchy folliculitis on my arms from a bad calving. Other than this spinal stress fracture I've had no actual veterinary-induced broken bones. I've got off quite lightly.

But a sore back should not have been a surprise. Some of it was self-inflicted. Years of pounding the streets of Castleford in my schooldays, stretching every sinew for those marginal gains in the weekend's cross-country race, had been the starting point. Mountain biking crashes, hiking and climbing up steep-sided mountains in the Alps, bent double by a huge rucksack full of climbing equipment. And the miles of triathlon training in my pursuit of Team GB success had not helped either. Neither had the thousands of kilometres of training for my world record indoor rowing in 2009, nor my recent habit of ski mountaineering racing.

I am not a brilliant skier, but I love being in the mountains and this, ironically, offered a (relatively) safe and a (relatively) non-concussive sport to keep me fit and sane. In 2018 I raced from Zermatt to Verbier in the famous Patrouille des Glaciers, a tough ski mountaineering race organised by the Swiss army. I'd entered in a team of three with two of my mates, Francesca and Dave, who both lived in the Alps and had snowy slopes and peaks on their doorsteps, while I had a ski machine in my garage. This is regarded as the hardest amateur endurance team event in the world (which is, obviously, why I decided I had to do it), and it covered fifty-three kilometres and about four and a half thousand metres of vertical height gain.

The race started at eleven o'clock in the evening and we gathered an hour beforehand in the dark, arranged in groups of a few hundred. There were nerves aplenty because everyone on the starting line knew what was in store for them over the next ten to fourteen hours. It was like the beginning of *The Hunger Games*, as we stood nervously awaiting our fate with hundreds of other optimistic sadists all dressed in weird Lycra suits, helmets and head-torches. I had to pinch myself. It seemed a million miles from the gentle grassy slopes of Yorkshire. The hooter went and our wave of 'Patrouilleurs' set off into the night and into a huge adventure. Three hours later, roped together, Francesca, Dave and I struggled up a steep, icy slope. We dared not contemplate a slip. It was a long way down the glacier, behind us in the blackness.

But we made it through, and the next day, in the blazing heat, we limped, exhausted and bedraggled, burnt and dehydrated, jubilant into Verbier. My legs were weary and, unbeknownst to me until much later, my back had suffered another major setback.

So, as I drove home from Mr Wilson's farm, I considered how many more calvings like this one I would be able to do. The pain was ebbing as the heat from my car seat eased into my stricken nerves and muscles. It was a strange thing to think that I might have to put this part of my life to one side, and I thought back over some of the most memorable deliveries which I had performed – mostly challenging, all rewarding and not all cold, wet and windy. Which reminded me . . .

One of the first was quite the opposite. Some heifers had been grazing on the rough grassland surrounding a huge country house. It was, in fact, the huge country house in which Donald Sinclair – aka Siegfried Farnon in the Herriot stories – had once lived. The heifers were enjoying the summer grazing and should not have been pregnant, but one had obviously had an illicit encounter with a bull. She had started to give birth but, because of her youth, had run into problems. The gardener had spotted the stricken heifer on the hillside while he was mowing the lawns and called the surgery. It was nearly lunchtime so, as the most junior vet, I was sent to solve the problem. In the warm sunshine, removing my shirt to reach inside the heifer was hardly work. The hard part had been catching her in a makeshift pen. The gardener and a villager who had been roped in to help seemed amazed at the whole process and, shortly after the calf was delivered, someone produced three small bottles of beer, which had been chilling in a nearby stream. Sitting on a sunny bank watching the new mother with her unexpected calf was pleasant enough, but to be able to enjoy a beer too was exceptional.

I rubbed my back again, grimacing for the umpteenth time. I would need the help of experts if I were to be able to continue with the work I loved. For once, my own grit and determination would not be sufficient. I would not be able to rely solely on my resilience and sense of duty towards the animals of Yorkshire. The next day, I was booked in to have a double epidural injection into my spine. I hoped it would work its magic and that it would not leave me as wobbly as Mr Wilson's cow!

To my disappointment, the pair of epidural injections, each bigger than the one I'd put into Mr Wilson's cow the night before, did not work any magic at all. After two weeks, I was back to discuss a treatment plan with the surgeon. For once, the patient did not have four legs. It had two and it was me. The spondylolisthesis and accompanying stress fracture had resulted in a hopelessly unstable base to my spine, the very bit of my anatomy that was supposed to provide the most rigid support. My backbone – the very essence both literally and metaphorically of solidity – was neither solid nor supporting.

Three weeks later, I sat on a hospital bed interrogating the anaesthetist about my pre-med. Then I had a long and involved discussion with the surgeon. Were the screws self-tapping or would he drill a guide hole, I asked, keen to know as much about the surgical process as I could. This thirst for the details disguised the fact that I was scared. This time someone else would be holding the scalpel.

Once in the pre-op room, I peered into theatre. There was another person where I would normally have been standing. I was the one about to be lying, asleep, on the table. I had no control and was relying on the skills of another surgeon. And then I knew how my animal patients might feel. For once, the next creature, neither great nor small, was me.

Acknowledgements

This, my most recent book, is also my biggest. It's taken longer to write than the others. I started grappling with a format before the completion of *The Next Chapter*, back in the autumn of 2019. It's hardly of Tolstoy proportions, but the pile of papers in front of me on the table as I compile this final and simplest section, is satisfyingly fat. *All Creatures* recollects past stories and anecdotes from the beginning of my life with animals right up to one of the final bovine pieces of surgery I've performed.

I'm grateful to Hannah Black, my editor at Hodder and Stoughton for the flexibility and freedom to "let me crack on". Your advice has been as invaluable as it has been unobtrusive. My literary agent, David Riding, possesses similar attributes – thank you, too.

Compiling these stories has been set against the backdrop of another professional change for me – the opening of, and move to, a new practice. At last my own and moulded in the way that Helen, Mark, Tracy and I wish. It's in its early stages, but the future is surely bright! Thank you to my new colleagues, who have borne the brunt of the challenges that opening a new practice brings. This book was also developed during the horrors of a pandemic, which has had an indelible impact on everyone's life. Writing about my animal anecdotes has been a huge positive during the dark days of "lockdown". I hope positivity exudes from the pages of this book to readers, too.

Ross Blair, my cameraman for *The Yorkshire Vet* over the last three years, has been a constant friend and companion, as quiet and perennial as a rock. It turns out he's a dab hand with a still camera, because he kindly took the cover shots for this book. Ian, of *Ian's Mobile Nanny Goat Farm*, kindly offered his animals for the cover picture – thank you for this and also for your help over the last year.

Thank you to the animal-owning public of Yorkshire, without whom these stories would not exist and thank you to Anne for yet more painstaking checking and metaphorical red pen in the margin!